ADHD IN ADULTS

Effective Strategies, Skills, And Self-Help To Improve the Quality of Life For Those Who Have It And Those Who Take Charge of a Loved One.

By
Diana Shelby

© Copyright 2021 – All rights reserved.

The content contained within this book may not be reproduced, duplicated, or transmitted without direct written permission from the author or the publisher.

Under no circumstances will any blame or legal responsibility be held against the publisher, or author, for any damages, reparation, or monetary loss due to the information contained within this book. Either directly or indirectly.

Legal Notice:

This book is copyright protected. This book is only for personal use. You cannot amend, distribute, sell, use, quote or paraphrase any part, or the content within this book, without the consent of the author or publisher.

Disclaimer Notice:

Please note the information contained within this document is for educational and entertainment purpose only. All effort has been executed to present accurate, up to date, and reliable, complete information. No warranties of any kind are declared or implied. Readers acknowledge that the author is not engaging in the rendering of legal, financial, medical, or professional advice. The content within this book has been derived from various sources. Please consult a licensed professional before attempting any techniques outlined in this book.

By reading this document, the reader agrees that under no circumstances is the author responsible for any losses, direct or indirect, which are incurred as a result of the use of the information contained within this document, including, but not limited to, errors, omissions or inaccuracies.

This book is a work of fiction. Any resemblance to actual person, living or dead, or actual events is entirely coincidental. Names, characters, businesses, organizations, places, events, and incidents are products of the author's imagination or are used fictitiously.

This information is not intended as a substitute for professional medical advice, emergency treatment or formal first-aid training. Do not use this information to diagnose or develop a treatment plan for a heath problem, disease or mental disturb without consulting a qualified health care provider. If you are in a life-threatening or emergency medical situation, seek medical assistance immediately.

Table of Contents

Introduction 6

1. Don't let ADHD turn your life upside down! 9

5 Effective Strategies for Adults with ADHD 9

2. ADD vs ADHD: What is the Difference? 17

The Most Common and Widespread Misconceptions 17

3. Cognitive Behavioral Therapy (CBT) in Adults with ADHD 23

4. Dopamine: The Motivational Molecule 26

5. ADHD Emotions: Watch Out for A Condition Called Rejection-Sensitive Dysphoria (RSD) 34

6. ADHD: Moments of Meltdowns 38

7. ADHD Is More Than What Others See from The Outside. 43

8. ADHD and Romantic Relationships 47

9. Love and ADD/ADHD 57

10. Tips and Strategies for Families With ADHD 64

11. ADHD and Eating Disorders 75

Foods to avoid. 75

12. Practice Mindfulness Meditation in ADHD 82

13. ADHD and Managing Finances 87

14. Strategies for Maintaining Focus If You Have ADHD 92

15. Myths to Dispel About Women And ADHD 102

16. The Positive Side Of ADHD: Creativity 106

17. A Direct and Moving Testimony............................110

18. The 12 Most Famous Personalities With ADHD ... 114

Final Thoughts 119

Introduction

Welcome and thank you for reading this book.

Before beginning, it is necessary to clarify what ADHD is, although it is implied that if your eyes have stopped on this book, you should already be quite familiar or fairly familiar with this topic and perhaps you are looking for some additional strategies or some simple tips to handle yourself or someone by your side.

ADHD stands for attention deficit hyperactivity disorder.

ADD stands for attention deficit disorder.

These disorders include difficulties with attention and concentration, impulse control, and activity level. They stem essentially from the child's inability first, and the adult in the future, to adapt his or her behavior according to the normal passage of time such as having a quiet daily routine, the goals to be achieved (of any kind) and the demands of the environment (from school to work, family, and so on).

ADHD is a real problem; but guess what? If there is a problem, there is also a solution.

It is a problem for the individual, for the family and for the context in which one live, and it is often an obstacle to achieving personal goals. It is a condition that frequently generates despair and stress also for those people who find themselves unprepared to manage with someone who has ADHD.

The disorders related to attention deficit disorder (ADD) or Attention Deficit Hyperactivity Disorder (ADHD) are due to an altered development of brain circuits that underlie important cognitive functions, including the capacity for sustained attention and control of instinctive motor responses. This disorder affects 3-4% of children and about 1% of adults. About one-third of children with this disorder continue to have problems after age 18. Indeed, it should be noted that in adults, the problems become more complex. The motor hyperactivity typical of the child is internalized and often manifests itself in anxiety disorders. The inability to plan daily activities or to be punctual in work or personal commitments, is often interpreted as lack of motivation or respect for others, sometimes causing irreparable relationship rifts.

In adults, attention disorders can cause significant problems in family and work relationships, especially if you are placed in a context where the disorder is not known or not understood. Often those affected find enormous difficulty in managing the activities of daily life, even the most ordinary as grabbing the phone to look for a contact in the phone book and then completely forget who wanted to call. There is also a problem of self-esteem and loss of confidence in their abilities. It is not uncommon for young people with this disorder to seek help after adolescence, very often in relation to difficulties they encounter when they begin college, their first romantic dates or a new job.

So, whatever your position right now, whether as a person with this disorder or as an acquaintance of a person with ADHD or ADD, I hope you will benefit from the pages that follow where we are going to look together at some effective strategies for living your best life.

1. Don't let ADHD turn your life upside down!

5 Effective Strategies for Adults with ADHD

Keeping track of a life of what was once a child and then a teenager with ADHD, can continue to be arduous and exceedingly difficult into adulthood.

Simple things that usually help us do our daily work, whether at home or in the office, are often not even considered for a person with ADHD. However, there is a way to try to find an easy passage through what might seem like a complicated maze, namely the mind of a person with ADD or ADHD.

Much research around the world highlights that targeted strategies can significantly help people with ADHD compensate for their deficits and have a more peaceful life.

In this chapter, we begin by looking at some of the most proven strategies that can come to the aid of adults with ADHD.

1. Strategy: Do You Have ADHD? Do You Have It or Not?

A wise first move to make in establishing a peaceful coexistence with ADHD is to be aware that you actually have ADHD. It sounds bizarre, but many adults are unaware of their condition. They sadly blame themselves or accept blame from those in their circle of affection for their lack of interpersonal skills and inadequate level of concentration.

Living in denial, or even ignorance, is a common practice among ADHD adults. Often these people fail to take note of the alarming signs of ADHD and continue to deny or discount their condition until test results, if not some profoundly serious occurrence, prove the exact opposite.

Detecting ADHD in adults, however, could be a challenge for even the best specialists. That is because the associated symptoms are quite similar to others related to other conditions, such as anxiety and depression, or particularly sensitive characters. Unlike anxiety and depression, which can occur quite often from the social and general stresses derived from adult life (relationships, employment, parenting, financial responsibilities, and so on), ADHD, on the other hand, is primarily a neurobiological disorder.

2. Strategy: Identify Problem Areas.

People with ADHD differ in their abilities and deficiencies. Every single human being in the world is in his or her own way unique and special as well as different from everyone else in personality, character, personal and family history, education level, background, and so on. You need to identify your personal problem areas in every sense of the word. Ask your specialist, then your family members, friends or why not your colleagues if you spend most of your day with them, to help you identify these problems. Once you have clarity, it is immensely helpful to compare notes with other adults with ADHD, listening to their experiences could be a great help and source of inspiration.

Further investigation should be done regarding a distinction between ADHD and ADD, but we will cover this in the next chapter.

3. Strategy: Getting Organized Across the Board.

Getting organized is among the most difficult challenges a person with ADHD faces, well, actually it is for a lot of people, but for them the difficulties are greater. Nevertheless, the best you can do is roll up your sleeves and find effective strategies to get organized!

You can start by learning how to break down a single task into small steps. To eat any dish what do we do? We take small doses at a time, take a bite, chew, and swallow, right? Well, the same should be done for organizing your daily routine as well. For example: why does the shopping list have to hang on the wall in the kitchen or on top of the refrigerator? Who said that? Let us assume you are at home, you walk into the bathroom and discover you are out of hand soap, or toothpaste, or shampoo. It would be difficult for any adult to keep in mind to add toothpaste to the shopping list once you leave the bathroom and return to the kitchen, let alone an adult with ADHD. If, on the other hand, we made sure we had a small list (just a piece of paper and a pencil, it is enough) even in the bathroom it would be much easier, wouldn't it? So, the message is this: focus on each step at a time. According to experts, this is a useful strategy that helps you complete the entire task, step by step, without getting discouraged by its size. With the completion of each step, a person gets motivated to move on to the next one.

Keeping a to-do list to compensate for the tendency to forget is a super simple and amazingly effective action. A detailed to-do list (on paper or on your phone) should contain everything you want to do that particular day, but also that week or even season by season. This operation should not be seen as a burdensome work, but rather as a valuable aid to recover your serenity. Imagine a visually impaired person wearing glasses, the same function more or less has to be that of lists for a person with ADHD.

Experts also point to the fact that making a list and being able to check off all the lines is like achieving small goals that over time will increase the confidence of ADHD patients. Experts also recommend using different colors as a background for the different tasks listed, for example, what pertains to family in green, business in blue, payment deadlines in red, and so on. Colors act as a strong mnemonic for an adult with ADHD.

Making lists and organizing each part of the day into portions will naturally and positively result in better time track keeping, which is another major challenge an adult with ADHD faces. A simple and easy way to keep track of time is get into the habit of checking the time. It could be remarkably effective to organize your day by listing what to do and how much time to spend on each activity already while you prepare your overall list. For example, you know that on Wednesday you will have to pick up laundry from the laundry room, attend a business meeting, and maybe go to a dinner party for the birthday of a friend you want to give a gift to.

Start by listing how much time the meeting will take up (including time to prepare any paperwork or red tape that may arise) and what part of the day it is scheduled for, then decide when to pick up the dry cleaning, and finally figure out if you will have time to stop at the mall to look for a gift to bring to your birthday friend or if you would be better off delegating the gift search or dry cleaning pickup to your partner or someone else. Try to stick to your plan. Use organizers and planners for your monthly or yearly plans and set reminders on your phone and computer.

4 Strategy: Balancing Diet and Exercise

You hear it everywhere and it is applicable to anyone, regardless of whether you have ADHD or not: a balanced diet and regular healthy exercise will reduce your stress level. No one expects you to become Rocky Balboa and start working out to exhaustion every day or to play sports if you hate playing sports. Exercise also means a walk outside on your lunch break, taking the stairs instead of taking the elevator, playing ball with kids if there are any, and other low impact activities. You may be skeptical, but a great tool for mindfulness and mental rebalancing is also meditation, perhaps combined with a gentle exercise or yoga session.

Finally, no one is talking about diets in the sense of banning particular foods like fats, sweet carbs, and so on. Only, in this case, the idea is to integrate a little bit of everything in your diet, clearly favoring healthy foods and rich in vitamins, lots of fruits and vegetables. Why not substitute a snack with an apple or a salad for chips? Maybe not always, once you do it one way once another. This can help you expand your attention span and increase blood circulation in your body.

5 Strategy: Determination and High Spirit

ADHD is a condition you live with every day, weekdays and holidays, day, and night. It is not something that can be interrupted or paused just at will like an episode of a TV show. For this reason, and for the simple fact that you are a human being with feelings and not a robot, it is more than normal that sometimes you might feel depressed, defeated, unlucky and unmotivated to improve things. Maybe you are maturing a good achievement of your goals, but sometimes it does not feel like enough. In these moments, you need to understand that it is all a consequence of ADHD symptoms and that they can disappear by consistently following the strategies set out above.

Always remember that you must overcome many more obstacles than someone without ADHD, and that involves having to be stronger and more determined. You need to keep yourself motivated by reminding yourself of your accomplishments/progress, even minimal ones. It is important to develop a good amount of self-love, self-esteem, and awareness. Talk to your family members and the people closest to you, ask them to support and encourage you in your efforts. It may even be that you do not need to ask, that if you pay attention, you will notice that those around you love and support you in spite of everything. So, ask yourself, isn't it worth it to improve and make those who love you proud of you?

Do not allow depressive states to crush you under their weight, this is a common tendency among adults with ADHD and it is critical to create a good defensive weapon for yourself.

As an adult, you are expected to manage your own life and there are many social responsibilities to take care of, for yourself and everyone around you, so grab your sword and shield and be stronger than you are. Do not let ADHD turn your life upside down!

2. ADD vs ADHD: What is the Difference?

The Most Common and Widespread Misconceptions

"Oh, please, I know you can't have ADHD dear...you're not hyper!" This is one of the most common misconceptions about attention deficit hyperactivity. The truth is that you can have the condition, even if you are not loud, impulsive, and you are not jumping around rooms.

People with ADHD are loud, outspoken, and physically active, right? No, this is an incorrect statement. Many people with ADHD, especially girls and women, live with a quiet form of the condition related to the disorder that is often misunderstood and undiagnosed. While hyperactivity is clearly impossible to ignore in children, adults who have trouble listening or are always late or are extremely distracted risk being seen as rude or "head-in-the-clouds" people. In the quiet forms, the symptoms of ADHD are never identified or treated. That's why it becomes very useful to identify the different variations of attention deficit.

What is ADHD?

As anticipated in the preceding pages, attention deficit hyperactivity disorder, ADHD, is the preferred medical term for the biologically based neurological condition once called ADD. Symptoms fall into three main categories: poor attention, poor impulse control, and sometimes hyperactivity. They also vary in type and severity from person to person, based on their gender and age, as well as, of course, each patient's personal history, making diagnosis difficult. The group of behaviors that make up ADHD have been recognized since 1902, although the name has changed over time. According to the Centers for Disease Control and Prevention, 9.5% of children and adolescents in the United States have been diagnosed with ADHD.

ADD vs ADHD.

ADHD is the official and most popular medical term for identifying the condition regardless of whether a patient exhibits symptoms of hyperactivity. ADD, on the other hand, is an obsolete term that is generally used to describe ADHD that has symptoms such as disorganization, lack of concentration, and forgetfulness.

Inattentive ADHD

Inattentive ADHD is often categorized as apathetic behavior in children, or depression/anxiety in adults. People with this form of ADHD often lose focus, are forgetful, and seem to have difficulty listening to anyone who comes to them. According to the Diagnostic and Statistical Manual of Mental Disorders-V (DSM-V), six of the following symptoms must be present and cause severe impact at school or work or in well-defined settings to merit a diagnosis.

- Often fails to pay attention to details or makes distracting errors.
- Often has difficulty with sustained attention.
- Often does not appear to listen when spoken to.
- Often does not follow instructions and fails to complete projects or tasks.
- Often has difficulty with tasks and organization activities.
- Often avoids or is reluctant to engage in tasks that require mental effort.
- Often loses things needed for tasks and activities and cannot remember where he left them.
- Is often easily distracted by extraneous stimuli, even minimal ones.
- Is often careless in daily activities.

This may sound like a strong statement, but it must be said that recognizing Inattentive ADHD is the key to avoiding a life of low self-esteem, messy relationships, and often shame.

The Hyperactive-Impulsive Type

The Hyperactive-Impulsive Type is the stereotype that most people picture someone to when they think of ADHD. A rowdy young boy who jumps around rooms, throws things everywhere, and interrupts others mid-sentence. However, this description fits only a small fraction of those with the condition. To have this type, a person must have 6 or more of the following symptoms:

- He or she fidgets with hands or feet or wiggles in a chair.
- In the case of a child or teenager, he or she is out of place in class or in other situations where he or she is expected to remain seated.
- Scurries and jumps everywhere excessively in situations where he or she is out of place (in adolescents or adults, this may be limited to subjective feelings of restlessness. In an adult, for example, it may be difficult to remain seated at the table during a meal or during any kind of long ceremony).

- He or she has difficulty playing or engaging in fun and entertainment in a quiet manner.
- Appears or acts as if he or she is "driven by a motor."
- Talks excessively instead of quietly engaging in what he or she is doing.
- Misplaces answers before questions have been completed.
- Has difficulty waiting his turn.
- Interrupts or meddles with others (intrudes in the middle of others' conversations or activities).

Combined Type ADHD

Combined type ADHD occurs when someone has 6 or more symptoms of inattention, and 6 or more symptoms of hyperactivity and impulsivity. Men and boys more commonly have hyperactive symptoms, while women and girls more commonly have inattention symptoms. Because of this, men are more commonly diagnosed than women, as their symptoms are more easily recognized as ADHD by both specialists and family members.

To avoid the continued spread of missed diagnoses, it is important that medical professionals learn to recognize all types of ADHD, as well as how some related conditions are often mistaken as ADHD, and that those who think they have or find themselves in a relationship with a person with the disorder take steps to treat the disorder.

3. Cognitive Behavioral Therapy (CBT) in Adults with ADHD

There is a lot of interest - but also apparently a lot of confusion - about the nature of cognitive behavioral therapy and how it can be used to help adults with ADHD. Cognitive behavioral therapy refers to a type of mental health treatment that focuses on thoughts and behaviors that occur "in the here and now." This approach differs from traditional forms of psychoanalytic and psychodynamic therapy, which include replaying and reprocessing childhood experiences that may have resulted in current emotional problems. One difference of CBT over these earlier therapies is that its goals and methods are explicitly stated and, therefore, can be adjusted for everyone.

CBT originated from a 'union of cognitive therapy developed in 1960 by Aaron Beck and popularized by Albert Ellis, and behavioral therapy, developed by B.F.Skinner, Joseph Volpe and others. Beck and Ellis believed that we all have automatic thoughts that occur as an immediate response to an event, situation, or other stimulus. These thoughts and cognitions can be helpful, leading to positive feelings and an effective coping strategy, or they can be negative and lead to feelings of depression or anxiety and maladaptive behavior. These negative thoughts usually form the basis of irrational beliefs and cognitive distortions. Some examples include:

- all-or-nothing, or black-and-white thinking, which gives rise to perfectionism.
- Selective focus on negative events and outcomes (overriding positive outcomes)
- Catastrophism, believing that a catastrophe will happen if something does or does not occur.
- Personalization, seeing oneself as the cause of a negative external event when one is not, in fact, personally responsible for it.

Therapy helps identify these irrational beliefs by challenging and consequently analyzing and denying them as they arise through discussion and home exercises, which typically include keeping a written record of thoughts.

Over the years, cognitive therapy has been expanded and modeled for the treatment of depression and many specific types of anxiety, including generalized anxiety disorder, social anxiety, post-traumatic stress disorder, and obsessive-compulsive disorder. Being attacked in treatment are negative behaviors, as well as negative thoughts (hence the term cognitive - behavioral therapy). Exercises in the session and at home typically include gradual and systematic exposure to triggering situations and the development and testing of skills to better manage these situations, as well as questioning the automatic and irrational thoughts that can often appear.

How is CBT relevant to adults with ADHD?

CBT is relevant to adults with ADHD in two ways.

First, in recent years, CBT programs have been developed specifically for adults with ADHD. Some of these programs aspire to help adults overcome their difficulties in the executive functions that are needed every day to effectively manage time, organize, and plan for the short and long term. Other programs focus on emotional self-regulation, impulse control, and stress management.

Programs that address executive dysfunction fall into the category of cognitive behavioral therapy because they impart more adaptive cognition about how to plan, organize, etc. and also more effective behavioral skills. An example of an adaptive cognition is the self-instruction of "reducing complex or unpleasant tasks into manageable parts." Examples of behavioral skills are using an agenda regularly and implementing a document categorization system. Positive thinking and positive behaviors reinforce each other. As stated earlier, as a person becomes more effective at managing time, he or she begins to have more positive beliefs and cognitions about him or herself and this in turn helps generate and maintain more adaptive behaviors.

4. Dopamine: The Motivational Molecule

What is dopamine?

Dopamine is a neurotransmitter critical for motivation, concentration, and productivity.

In the human brain there are almost 100 billion neurons, (almost the same number as the stars in the Milky Way just to give you an idea!) and these cells communicate with each other through substances called neurotransmitters, among them dopamine gives us motivation, drive, and concentration. A sort of personal cheerleader.

It is often called the molecule of motivation precisely because it stimulates our determination and concentration, making us keep the focus on the goals, giving us the necessary boost. It allows us to plan for the long term and resist distractions so that we can achieve our goals; in short, it gives us the support of the classic "*I got it!*" that we are used to saying when we achieve what we set out to do. It makes us more competitive and gives us the thrill of challenge in many aspects of our lives: work, sports, and love.

Dopamine is responsible for our reward system and allows us to experience feelings such as joy, bliss and even euphoria. Levels that are too low can make us unfocused, unmotivated, lethargic, and in severe cases, depressed.

What are Dopamine Deficiency Symptoms?

People with low levels of dopamine are immediately noticeable: they have little vitality and show little energy and motivation, so they often make excessive use of caffeine, sugar, or other stimulants of different types to get through the day. Some of the most common symptoms of Dopamine deficiency are quite similar to those of depression:

- Low motivation.
- Perennial fatigue.
- Apathy in all circumstances.
- Procrastination of any activity.
- Difficulty feeling pleasure.
- Low libido.
- Sleep disorders.
- Mood swings.
- Memory lapses.
- Difficulty concentrating.

In laboratory tests, the guinea pigs had become so apathetic and lethargic that they lost the drive to eat to the point of allowing themselves to starve. Conversely, some people with low levels of Dopamine tend to compensate with self-destructive behaviors that increase its levels, including use and abuse of caffeine, alcohol, sugar, energy drinks, drugs, shopping, extreme challenges, video games, uninhibited sex or dangerous sexual practices, gambling and more.

So, the question arises: **how to increase the levels with natural methods?**

There are plenty of unhealthy ways to increase dopamine levels, but you do not necessarily have to resort to "sex, drugs, and rock 'n' roll" to boost them. Here are some proven healthy methods that will allow you to increase your levels naturally. The advice, however, in this case as in general for any other topic covered in this book, remains to consult doctors and specialists, because each of us has different needs, so everything should be tailored.

Through the power of food. We are what we eat.

Dopamine is made up of the amino acid tyrosine. Following a diet rich in tyrosine-containing foods will provide you with the "batteries" you need to have optimal dopamine production. What are these foods?

- All foods of animal origin.
- Almonds.
- Apples.
- Avocados.
- Bananas.
- Beets.
- Chocolate.

- Coffee.
- Broad beans.
- Green leafy vegetables.
- Green tea.
- Lima beans.
- Oatmeal.
- Seaweed.
- Sesame and pumpkin seeds.
- Turmeric.
- Watermelon.
- Wheat germ.

In addition, foods high in probiotics like yogurt, kefir (aka the drink of centenarians!) and raw sauerkraut can naturally increase dopamine production. It may sound strange, but the health of your gut flora also affects neurotransmitter production. An overabundance of bad bacteria can release toxic byproducts called lipopolysaccharides that lower dopamine levels. Sugar can also increase its production, but this is a temporary effect that can be likened more to pharmacology than nutrition.

Through exercise.

Already in previous chapters I have emphasized how physical activity is one of the best aids a person can give to their brain and again I want to reiterate that. Exercise increases the production of new brain cells, slows down cellular aging, and increases the influx of nutrients to the brain. It can also increase your levels of dopamine and other "feel-good" neurotransmitters such as serotonin and norepinephrine.

Dr. John Ratey noted psychiatrist and author of the book "Spark: The revolutionary New Science of Exercise and the Brain" has extensively studied the effects of exercise on the brain and found that motor activity tends to raise baseline levels of dopamine, promoting the growth of new brain receptors. Dopamine is partly responsible for the performance of professional runners, but that does not mean you have to train hard to boost your brain. You do not need to become a frequent gym-goer, just take more walks in the fresh air (half an hour or as much as you can on your lunch break for example, if not in your free time) or more calm and focused physical activities such as yoga, can bring enormous benefits to your body-mind system.

With meditation.

The benefits of meditation are proven by an impressive number of professional studies, and it is now difficult to find people who show skepticism about meditation. Those who regularly practice meditation have increased their learning abilities, creativity, and relaxation. Meditation has been shown to increase dopamine, improving attention, one's balance and inner awareness and ability to concentrate.

The most appropriate type of meditation for those with ADHD is Mindfulness Meditation.

Manual hobbies of all kinds.

Knitting, sewing, drawing, chess, photography, woodworking, and DIY increase brain focus on much the same way as meditation. These activities increase dopamine levels, staving off depression and protecting against mental aging.

Listening to music.

Music, in any genre, can put dopamine into your bloodstream and, oddly enough, it seems that just the intention to listen is enough to allow it to be released.

Dopamine works as a sort of survival mechanism, releasing energy when we are faced with a great opportunity and rewarding us when our needs have been met. But be careful not to become obsessed with it, otherwise you risk becoming addicted to states of euphoria, greed, and lust that over time turn into something toxic.

Our ancestors, who lived a perpetual challenge for survival, consequently had a dopamine rush every time they found a new source of drinking water or a better place to hunt because it meant they could survive one more day and better. Although today you only need to go to the supermarket or stop at a diner to get food, there are definitely healthy ways to enjoy the sense of challenge even in this day and age. For example, you can reach a new professional goal, realize a dream in your drawer such as writing a book or opening a blog, close a difficult negotiation or even do something more pleasant and simple such as listening to new music or experimenting with special ingredients to cook with. If you share a common passion with your partner or friends, it can be exciting to plan a special trip perhaps to exotic places, look for a hard-to-find collector's item or the perfect gift for the person you care about. You can start hobbies based on achieving specific goals such as, for example, rock climbing, bird watching, collecting all kinds of items....

The act of seeking and finding always activates your reward mechanisms, without any kind of regret.

Create long-term and short-term goals for yourself, depending on the scope of the goal. Clearly you cannot set the goal of becoming a great cook in a week, you must try, experiment, fail and do it again, but maybe in a week you can finish that exceptionally long book that has been gathering dust on the nightstand next to your bed for too long.

If dopamine is released when we reach a goal, then setting only long-term goals can be frustrating and counterproductive, so try to set both near-term and longer-term goals. As mentioned, short-term ones do not have to be goals that are too challenging: finish a book, clean out a drawer, or take that trip just out of town that you never accomplished. Try to break down your more distant goals into a series of smaller steps so that you can self-help yourself with dopamine "boosts" along the way.

Above all, challenge yourself!

5. ADHD Emotions: Watch Out for A Condition Called Rejection-Sensitive Dysphoria (RSD)

ADHD, with its emotions and bringing everything into turmoil, can undermine self-esteem, relationships and have often irreparable consequences on almost everything else in life. Here is what you should know to better control that fragile part of every human being called emotionality.

Researchers have unfortunately ignored the emotional component of ADHD for too long because it cannot be measured. Yet, emotional dysfunction represents the most negative aspects of ADHD at any age and for any gender.

Sensitive to criticism.

Nearly all individuals with diagnosed ADHD answer an emphatic yes to the question, "Have you always been more sensitive than others to rejection, feeling teased, criticism, or your own perception that you have failed or are about to fail? ". This is the definition of a condition called rejection-sensitive dysphoria (RSD), which many individuals with ADHD experience personally.

Depression and RSD (rejection-sensitive dysphoria).

For many years, RSD has been the hallmark of what is called atypical depression. The reason it has not been called "typical" depression is that it is not depression at all, but the ADHD nervous system's instantaneous response to the rejection trigger.

Disapproval from others.

The emotional response to failure is truly catastrophic for those experiencing the condition. The criticism, perceived lack of affection and respect are just as devastating as if they were real. The term "dysphoria" means "hard to bear" and most people with ADHD report that they "can hardly bear it." People with ADHD are not shy, but disapproval harms them far more than it does neurotypical people.

Always tense as violin strings.

Many ADHDs say the same thing when you ask them about their emotional life: "*I'm always tense, I can never relax. I cannot sit there and watch a TV show with the rest of the family. Because I am sensitive to other people's disapproval of me, I fear personal relationships.*" Most children after the age of 14, do not show very obvious hyperactivity, but this is still present internally.

How suffering is expressed.

If emotional suffering is internalized, a person with ADHD may experience depression and loss of self-esteem in a short time, with even profoundly serious consequences. If emotions are externalized, grief may be expressed as anger toward a person or situation that has hurt them. Fortunately, in most cases anger is expressed verbally rather than physically, and this passes relatively quickly, although dragging with it a kind of latent repentance.

ADHD emotions: locked in a shell.

Because of sensitivity to emotional distress, the person may become a pleasant person, always making sure that friends, acquaintances, and family approve of him: *"tell me what you want, and I'll do my best to get it. Just don't get mad at me."* After years of constant vigilance, the ADHD person becomes a chameleon who loses track of what they want for their life. Some people with ADHD find that the pain of failure is so intense that they refuse to try anything unless they are assured of quick, easy, and complete success. A try is too great an emotional risk. Their lives remain stunted and limited, locked in a shell.

RSD (rejection sensitive dysphoria) can devastate relationships.

Since RSD injuries are almost unbearable for a person with ADHD, the only way to cope is to deny that the person, who may be a teacher, responder, relative, co-worker, or spouse, who is rejecting, criticizing, or teasing matters in the ADHD person's life. So instead of suffering at the hands of an authority figure, their importance is devalued. People with ADHD, several times a day, find opportunities to remind the other person how useless, stupid, and even harmful they and their opinions are.

6. ADHD: Moments of Meltdowns

Meltdowns are moments of more or less dramatic crisis that happen to any person, but when this touches an adult person with ADHD, it is almost inevitable that issue becomes a lot more delicate to manage.

Unfortunately, very often meltdowns are seen as simple moments of hyperactivity or misunderstood as attempts to grab attention or anything similar, on the contrary it is something extremely more complex.

In most cases, the experience of a meltdown for a person with ADHD involves moments of severe public embarrassment, the consequences of which are then felt, moments of extreme vulnerability, total unpredictability, and a kind of blind rage.

In the vast majority of cases, meltdowns are due to strong stress, emotional accumulation or repressed feelings, overstimulation of the senses, and in the worst-case scenario, a combination of several factors. When a meltdown is coming, it is exceedingly difficult to come out of it successfully. The best thing for people with ADHD is to first become aware of the trigger and note it in their diary or work journal. Alongside the triggering factor, it is a good idea to write down what happened during the moment of the collapse and how one felt just before the moment of reaching the point of no return.

In addition to this, it is important to understand how you were mentally and physically at the time of the breakdown. For example: had I slept the night before? Was I hungry or had I missed a meal? Had I received any bad news that day?

After all, a meltdown is a response to intense emotional activity triggered by an overwhelming situation. It is a moment comparable to when a wave that is too high, or too powerful, sweeps over a surfer on his or her run. Even the most experienced surfer will go underwater and lose control of himself for a few moments, in that moment, it is total darkness.

Typically, a meltdown involves:

- Excessive crying.
- Shaking.
- Throwing or breaking anything that comes near.
- Screaming (often includes swearing).
- Severe heart palpitations.
- Kicking and punching.

As already mentioned, the ideal is to learn how to manage the triggers (may be deadlines at work, economic difficulties, love relationships, a particularly cruel and intrusive person, and so on) jotting them down in a diary, even a note on the phone is fine, the important thing is that it is always updated, and completing the report with causes and consequences.

Example:

Date: June 1, 2021

Meltdown

Trigger:

Premenstrual dysphoric disorder (PMDD). Extreme mood swings, irritability, difficulty sleeping.

What happened:

I broke down crying in the office in front of colleagues.

Consequences:

Sadness, shocked faces, need to justify and horrible feeling of being subjected to public embarrassment.

If I ever find myself overwhelmed by this factor again, how can I avoid meltdown:

Do something that usually feels better to me. Phone my best friend, listen to that lovely song, get away from my desk and take a walk outside.

Then, it is good to try to plan a possible reduction of stress at the base of the excess of tension, find more time for recreation, and practice meditation activities that lead to greater attention to self-awareness.

Finally, it is always a good thing to remember not to skip meals, get enough rest, exercise (great if done outdoors), and to keep yourself constantly hydrated by avoiding drinks containing caffeine or too much sugar.

Instead, people who witness a meltdown of a person with ADHD may find other types of suggestions helpful, such as:

- ask before launching into hugs or caresses, they may not be appreciated.
- Be calm and patient.
- Let them know you are there, without being intrusive.
- Identify any triggers and remove them (if possible).
- Do not ask too many questions or complicated questions.
- Do not get all psychology-y on me or say chocolaty things.
- If you are within the walls of the house, it is useful to create a calming environment: close the curtains, turn off any source of noise or light such as TV, PC, alarm clocks, radio and do not force a person to leave the room chosen as a refuge.

- Do not flee in the face of an impending meltdown or a person in the process of meltdown.

Most importantly, never judge or judge yourself, and let things settle without forcing.

The key is patience and gentleness.

7. ADHD Is More Than What Others See from The Outside.

Both in cases of adults who have not yet been diagnosed with ADHD, and in cases of people who have someone with an ADHD condition around them, as mentioned in the other chapters it can happen that so many situations are misunderstood or mishandled.

In particular, where hyperactivity is not as obvious and visible, it is more likely to fall into conflict. For some individuals it has been lifesaving to have a diagnosis of ADHD to understand the causes of bouts of hyper focus, compulsive shopping, mood swings, and so on. It is worthwhile, therefore, to empty the bag and make it truly clear that most people with ADHD have these symptoms in common or have been in certain situations, hoping that this will be helpful both from those "in it" and for those "seeing from the outside."

It is often clear from the outside that they are present:

frequent distractions

Hyperactivity (difficulty sitting, prolonged activity, and other experiences previously reviewed)

But what does not appear to everyone and often only to those experiencing ADHD is:

- Depression.
- Improper focusing nor hyper focusing.
- Estrangement from reality.
- Rejective Sensitive Dysphoria (of which I have already covered)
- Auditory processing disorder.
- Repression of emotions.
- Exhausting lack of rest and difficulty in getting to sleep.
- Difficulty in finding the true nature of themselves because it is often preferred to wear "masks" to try to blend better in the crowd.
- Often the hyperactivity that is not seen from the outside is all in the mind, where total chaos reigns. Tangled thoughts, uncontrollable flows of emotions, mad airplanes, magicians and jugglers, acrobats, and parallel worlds (metaphorically speaking).
- There are times when everything seems really hard to manage, and simple things like one's job, one's role in the family (husband or wife, parent, child and so on) seems untenable, one's social status, people's expectations and even one's hobbies or goals.
- Difficulty or fear of asking for help, even from family and close friends.

- Constant feeling of guilt if you are not doing anything productive, even triggering paranoia while trying to rest.
- It is not always easy to accept yourself as you are, beyond the mood swings, some days are better and others everything seems to fall apart.
- It becomes almost traumatic to be labeled by those unfamiliar with ADHD as "a daydreamer creative type".
- They often fear that people around them will not accept them or will grow tired of them.
- Perennial terror of others' judgment.
- Attempts to produce dopamine by means that are sometimes harmful and dangerous to themselves and others: compulsive shopping for shiny things, eating disorders, and more.

Understanding everything listed in the lines above can take years and years of patience and study. Often it is not possible to do it alone, it is necessary, and especially recommended not to say indispensable, to turn to one or more professionals: psychologists, nutritionists, psychiatrists, therapists.

Please, never allow yourself to suffer alone or allow someone dear to you to plough a stormy sea without sharing and a life preserver to cling to.

8. ADHD and Romantic Relationships

I decided to dedicate this chapter to all lovers, because ADHD is an often underestimated or undiscussed problem when it comes to love and romantic relationships.

Below I will attempt to address the topic by giving suggestions for both those who experience ADHD as an affected person and as someone involved in a relationship.

Very frequently it is girls who do not know how to approach an involvement with a guy with ADHD, and that is why I will start with that. However, the same suggestions apply to any type of couple regardless of sexual gender.

Ask in a gentle way, never intrusively, as ADHD makes him or her feel.

Those without ADHD do not understand or have a hard time empathizing with the struggles of those with ADHD. Adults with this disorder often report that it is "they feel like their head is constantly disheveled by the wind, while they would like to maintain a good coiffure." Therefore, giving your fiancé a chance to open up and reveal how he or she is feeling can be very helpful and beneficial to both of you. Once you understand his feelings, it will be easier to offer support in a more constructive way.

Extremely important at this stage is to listen and never, ever put yourself in an attitude of disparagement or judgment.

Separate the person from the symptoms.

Let's take an example. Your boyfriend holds an important place in your life; he is a special person, right? Of course, therefore, he deserves to be treated in a special way. At times, ADHD symptoms can demean him, even lead him to dramatic meltdowns or to wearing masks that do not belong to him in order to hide the storm raging inside him, but all of these episodes should not be equated with him or your relationship. Never feel superior or put yourself in competition with ADHD symptoms. The mental and relational health of both partners involved is at stake. As he gains the tools to manage his symptoms, with the help of a professional and perhaps even the support of his girlfriend, the impact of the disorder on your life as a couple will lessen.

In the worst of times, it is helpful to remember the things that initially captivated and made you fall in love with that person.

Try to be a point of reference for him or her.

It is not easy nor something that can be learned in a short time, but it is essential to become able to recognize the most serious and compromising situations. Among these, the most common are a crowded place, with loud music and many people talking to each other at the same time, a mixture of smells ranging from deodorants, flowers, and food to perfumes and essences, and even a variety of light and flashing effects, such as those transmitted by the television or computer monitor. Overwhelming situations can generate a sense of oppressive feeling in an individual with ADHD. One solution to handling such situations is to act as a lifeline, a safe haven, during these episodes.

Being able to interpret his or her state of mind means knowing without delay when he or she will need to step outside for a moment and take a walk to calm down and ease his or her nerves.

Suggest and entice him to see a mental health professional.

Generally, adults with ADHD benefit tremendously from psychotherapy. This treatment helps them accept who they are and, at the same time, try to improve their situation.

During sessions, it is possible to address some of the fundamental problems caused by this disorder, such as time management and organization issues.

Look him in the eye when you talk to him.

Returning to the example of having a boyfriend. Help him focus and listen to your requests or continue the topic you are talking about through eye contact. Small gestures of seemingly harmless physical contact, such as a caress on the forearm or gently squeezing his hand as you talk to him, can help him keep his attention on what you are saying.

Do not touch his stuff.

In general, no one appreciates anyone else, from their parents to their partners, touching their things, but even more so and often, people with ADHD have a strong need to have all their belongings in a specific order or place. It is not a simple tendency to be habitual or a mania, sometimes it is a real lifeline to try to have a peaceful life. In the previous chapters we have often talked about strategies such as making lists, following a routine, putting keys and other easily lost items (glasses, earphones, pencils, etc.) always in the same place in order to facilitate finding them. Therefore, if, for example, in the evening he demands that his briefcase remain in a certain place, perhaps leaning against the last step of the staircase at the entrance or hanging from the door handle, do not move it. If you put it in another place because you do not like it or do not think that position is correct, know that he will almost certainly forget the briefcase at home, have problems at the office and you will have arguments over it. Habits allow people with ADHD to manage this disorder effectively, so do not mess up or meddle with these attempts.

Help him get organized.

As analyzed above, ADHD sufferers often have major problems with organization and time management. This can be a particularly frustrating aspect for those who do not have the syndrome. For example, if your boyfriend is forgetful or shows up late for appointments, help him get more organized by talking to him frequently about your schedule and keeping an updated calendar. Do not attack him as if it is personal or by misunderstanding that he does not care about the relationship, it is ADHD's fault (of course there are always exceptions). Having a diary or chalkboard hanging in the house or reminding him via a phone message, card, or other expedient (it depends a lot on habits, if the person who needs to be notified never looks at the phone, it will obviously be useless to send a text message) that you have an engagement, dinner, or anniversary, will greatly benefit the relationship.

Be prepared for mood swings.

Your boyfriend may be prone to mood swings that are sometimes sudden and indecipherable. Only by knowing what to do and how to react in such situations will you be able to calm him down. You should never feel guilty for an emotional dip or an outburst of anger, just stay close to your loved one by doing what is usually helpful in bringing him back in a good mood. Help him find something to distract him, turn on some music, tell a funny joke, or try to talk to him nicely.

Avoid Parenting.

One of the biggest challenges in a relationship with a partner with ADHD is the tendency to feel pressured to take charge. Since an individual with this syndrome has difficulty managing time, being organized, and maintaining focus, it is very likely that someone who doesn't have ADHD will want to take charge of everything. Or feel uncomfortable not doing so, not contributing. However, this behavior can trigger stress and resentment within the couple.

Speak up to communicate how you feel. Communicate to your partner how you feel, unfiltered, but be sure to emphasize that you take responsibility for your reactions so that you do not blame them. For example, you might say, "I feel like I have too much on my plate right now and can't get anything done. Could you please arrange to take the car to the mechanic?"

Divide up errands and cleaning according to your respective strengths and habits. Avoid disheartening yourself by choosing household chores that are more in line with your abilities and make it the same for your partner. For example, you could take charge of paying the bills and doing the weekly grocery shopping (remembering that for people with ADHD managing their own financial resources can prove to be a struggle), while your partner can take care of mowing the lawn or vacuuming.

Do not take things too personally and do not put yourself in the middle.

Your boyfriend is likely to have fits of nerves, engage in impulsive behaviors and be careless. As a result, you may feel unloved, offended, undervalued, or disregarded. However, keep in mind that he intentionally does nothing to fuel these feelings in you. ADHD prevents you from controlling certain behaviors, or more accurately, distorts your awareness. He can learn techniques that allow him to adapt to situations but try not to take his overreactions personally. Remember that ADHD is a real disease that goes into modifying behaviors.

Take care of yourself.

Recharge your batteries every once in a while. Living closely with someone with ADHD can be exhausting. It's bound to happen that you feel disheartened by all the support you're giving your partner. Therefore, consider it essential to take a break sometime so that you can regain your energy. For example, try having coffee alone, take up a hobby, or go to the movies with a friend.

Consult a psychotherapist, if possible, you can probably rely on the same professional who follows your partner. Psychotherapy can allow you to vent your frustrations in a healthy way and deal with problems with the help of trained guidance. Find a therapist who specializes in relationship problems and ADHD.

Finally, you can join the many organizations that allow people who are in relationships (of any kind) with individuals with ADHD to connect with each other and meet online or in person to share problems and solutions. Sometimes all it takes is a joke or a chat with someone who utterly understands, to feel comforted.

After this brief excursion, I would like to conclude that one of the worst causes of failure in relationships involving one or two individuals with ADHD is boredom. We already normally live in a world where we are constantly driven to seek new stimuli, new challenges and meet new people, but for an individual with ADHD, constant involvement and enriching the relationship with activities to do together with the partner is essential. This sounds absurd and unbelievable to someone who does not suffer from ADHD, but testimonies report of people ruining relationships simply because they forget to have relationships. Or of people getting involved in negative situations simply because of misdiagnosis or lack of communication.

Doing activities together, clearly related to one's customs, habits, and preferences, is extremely useful in facilitating dialogue and confrontation. Good activities are for example: swimming, dancing together, hiking, or long walks, trying new foods and exotic restaurants, playing a new game, competitions such as who can keep a plant from dying, watching movies and so on.

ADHD fortunately is not associated with any higher incidence of sexual disorders. But research has found more problems instead with sexual behavior. An earlier onset of sexual intercourse (during adolescence) and an overall riskier pattern to their sexual activity (more casual partners and less use of contraception) has been found.

This behavioral pattern is almost 10 times greater in being involved in a teenage pregnancy, as a father or mother (38% for the ADHD group versus 4% for the control group). There was also a 4-fold higher risk of having sexually transmitted diseases by age 20 (17% versus 4%).

The higher risk of becoming a parent in adolescence, when they are not yet able to raise a child, increases the subsequent likelihood of placing children for adoption, or having their children raised by their own parents (the child's grandparents) or by outsiders (babysitters, housekeepers).

As daunting as these various risks may seem, they can also serve to motivate young adults with ADHD to seek specialized, professional help.

9. Love and ADD/ADHD

Let us start by saying again that loving a person, affectionate, being in a relationship, is not easy at all. While it is the most natural thing in the world, I challenge you to find a single couple in the world that has never had to face difficulties (of any kind and regardless of gender, age, and characteristics of the components). Loving someone with ADD/ADHD, however, presents situations that test any person's limits.

Whether it is your child, boyfriend, girlfriend, partner, or spouse, it is important to learn how to cope with everyday life with them and to recognize the traits of this disorder. Understanding how a person with ADHD feels will help you become more patient, tolerant, compassionate, and loving towards them. Only by understanding ADHD will you have the keys to your loved one's heart. That is why I have decided to devote an additional chapter to this topic, and amplify the list of pointers, suggestions, or strategies - all terms are fine here - for dealing with a relationship situation.

Things to Remember.

They have an always-on mind. There is no on/off switch. There are no brakes that bring it to a halt. This is a burden that you must learn to manage.

- They listen, but do not absorb what is being said to them. As they say, it goes in one ear and out the other. A person with ADHD will look at you, appear to be listening to your words, but after a few minutes their mind is already on the road. They can still hear you talking, but their thoughts are now lost in space, in another galaxy.
- They have difficulty staying on the assigned task. Instead of keeping their attention on what they are doing, they distract themselves by staring at the colors on a wall in the room or what is hanging there. All it takes is a little bird outside the window or a dog barking in the distance.
- They become anxious quite easily and, like all deep thinkers, are extremely sensitive to everything that happens around them, both good and bad.
- They cannot concentrate when they are emotionally distracted. If there is something troubling going on, a person with ADHD cannot think about anything else. It is true that it happens to everyone, some more and some less, but in them this dynamic is more intense.
- In them, all emotions are amplified as if they were vibrations.
- They have difficulty interrupting the flow of emotions. Even when they are overwhelmed to the

point of almost extricating themselves from reality, they do not re-emerge.
- They have difficulty in regulating their emotions and even more often they are unable to contain them. The tangled threads in their hyperactive brains make thoughts and feelings difficult to separate, as if they were intertwined.
- They have verbal outbursts and intense emotions that they cannot regulate, and since they impulsively say what they think, they often say things that they later regret or repent, falling into a kind of self-guilt.
- For the above reason they suffer from social anxiety. They are afraid of saying something silly or reacting inappropriately. They often hold back from expressing themselves, so they feel safer, but this makes them much more anxious.
- They are deeply intuitive. They seem to possess an edge. ADHDers are often creatives, inventors, artists, musicians… This is a nice aspect.
- Another wonderful and often surprising facet of ADHD is that by thinking differently, their abstract minds see solutions to problems that others cannot.
- Never forget, however, that they are impatient and restless individuals. They are easily annoyed, wanting things to happen immediately.

- They are also physically hypersensitive. Insect bites like mosquito bites feel itchier. Even food or an environment can irritate them by taste or a simple smell if it is too impactful.
- A already seen in other chapters, they are totally disorganized. Accumulation is their preferred method of organization. Once a task has been completed, related papers or materials are placed in a corner where other piles of papers, clothing, objects, or things are stacked... Until the person with ADHD is overwhelmed or yelled at by someone and with great frustration then cleans up. It is difficult for a person with ADHD to keep things in order because their brain does not function in an orderly fashion.
- They need to move around, pretty much all the time. When they are talking on the phone maybe they walk around their desk, or they prefer to listen to an audiobook while walking around instead of reading stay sit it in their chair. Movement is a calming, soothing balm for them that brings clarity to their thoughts.
- Whenever they can, they avoid tasks that contain performance demands, especially if they are tied to a delivery time. Not because they are lazy or irresponsible, but because their minds are full of

options, possibilities and choosing is more problematic for them.
- They have difficulty remembering simple tasks. Another paradoxical feature of ADHD is in fact memory. People with ADHD cannot remember to shop for groceries for the week or buy a birthday card for a loved one, call the person they had an appointment with or even get to that appointment... but at the same time, they perfectly remember every comment, quote, or detail such as the number of victims of an accident they heard about on the radio. No matter how many reminders on the calendar they set, their distracted mind is always elsewhere. Undoubtedly, visible items (pictures) are easier for them to remember. That is why they have fifteen windows open on their desktop and a thousand screenshots saved in their phone's gallery.
- They carry on perhaps multiple tasks/engagements together because of the constant activity in their minds but, once one task is finished, they move on to the next without closing the previous task.
- They are passionate about anything that creates emotion or pleasure. Thoughts, words, behaviors of a person with ADHD are amplified and they give their heart and soul when they believe in something or have a feeling. In essence, a person with

ADD/ADHD, who we know has difficulty controlling their impulses, is a blessing if they channel their activities and emotions correctly. Perhaps, this is the quality and uniqueness that most makes them lovable and extraordinary people.

Sensitivity and a huge dose of patience will be essential to get through the most difficult times of living with a person with ADD or ADHD.

It is important, in the meantime, to take special care of yourself as well, taking regular personal time to collect your thoughts or participating in support groups for family members, getting informed, documenting, or even just venting to a wise, compassionate friend, finding time to pursue your hobbies and passions. In short, you should never forget to "unplug" from time to time.

We now know that some of the greatest inventors, artists, musicians, entrepreneurs, and writers had ADD/ADHD and probably were successful because they had a loved one who lovingly/unknowingly supported them in their daily struggles.

Therefore, they will have to learn how to manage anger and replace it with understanding, taking into account that it is not easy for them to comply with the behavioral expectations that society requires of them.

It must be admitted, people with ADD/ADHD are not easy to love, but utterly understanding the burden they also carry could be the key to living with it with more serenity.

10. Tips and Strategies for Families With ADHD

The latest statistics reveal that about 4% of adults in the United States have ADHD. Most of those affected are not diagnosed, nor are they receiving adequate treatment. This is likely due in part to the fact that ADHD in adults was not widely recognized until the mid-1980s, and before then this condition was really misunderstood. Since that moment, researchers have found that adults with ADHD are at risk for significant problems in their lives, in part because they often suffer from other disorders, such as anxiety and depression in addition to their ADHD.

Keeping in mind that ADHD is highly genetic and that there is about a 50% chance that an adult with ADHD will have one or more children with ADHD, it is no wonder that families with multiple ADHD members tend to have high levels of stress, marital conflict, and find parenting is a daunting responsibility.

Let us briefly consider once again what are the most common symptoms seen in adults and children with ADHD:

- Inattention.
- Hyperactivity/impulsivity.
- Distractibility.
- Forgetfulness.

- Problems with procrastination.
- Difficulty finishing tasks / projects.
- Emotional lability.

When both children and adults share the symptoms of ADHD, it becomes extremely difficult and challenging for all family members involved. For example, how does a distracted parent keep a child inattentive on task? How does a disorganized parent teach organizational strategies to children? How does a high-explosive parent tend to overstimulate a child? Imagine an adult with ADHD intent on helping a child with ADHD prepare an important assignment for a school exam, a pretty explosive picture emerges.

The adult with ADHD faces the already formidable task of raising an inherently stimulated child while simultaneously trying to cope with their own personal struggles. If the parents' ADHD issues are not addressed, they will find it extremely difficult to fulfill their role as effective parents. The specific needs of each individual family member, must be met in order for the family to manage effectively.

Listed below are some strategies deemed specific to use for those families who feel moved to want to improve relationships, self-esteem, and their family life in general.

Family strategies for living successfully with ADHD:

- Explicit help from partner and teamwork.
- Knowing that ADHD is part of the family traits, begin to change about expectations of yourself and your child. Expect that there will be more chaos, disorganization, and tension in your home and that everything will not be perfect like in the movies.
- Get help from a babysitter or relative or trusted person even if you are home, and possibly hire a competent person to do homework with your child. This will immediately lower the stress level for the entire family.
- Take parenting classes to acquire specific parenting tools.
- Realize that suggestions from friends and relatives, although intentional to help, may work for their children or life partners (who do not have ADHD), but not for you or your loved ones.
- Make sure that both parents' ADHD and the child's ADHD are treated optimally.
- Give yourself time when you feel you are about to lose control of yourself; teach your child to use the same tactics as you. Ask your spouse to take charge when

you feel overwhelmed and do not lose self-awareness. If you feel it helps, practice some controlled breathing exercises.

- Simplify your life in all areas: learn to say THANK YOU, but NO; or get in the habit of responding to outside requests by saying "I'll think about it and get back to you." This tactic forces you to think carefully about commitment before diving into an unsafe hole and perhaps crashing to the bottom. Stop before you have compromised.
- Delegate chores to each family member according to roles, do not charge everything onto your shoulders.
- Spend time with each child where the focus is solely on FUN.
- Learn to see the positive traits in all family members and remember to make them explicit by verbalizing them often, such as "hey your laughter cheers me up" or "the dinner you cooked was delicious."
- Spend time with your partner, friends, or even alone when you need to recharge: go to the movies, too see a concert, watch a sports game, or take a walk outside, whatever you like to do.
- Get help from a professional organizer to improve the systems already in place. Often, children and adults with ADHD do not have a natural understanding of

organizational methods; a professional organizer can be extremely helpful in teaching these strategies.

- Consider finding a good ADHD coach to help you prioritize, manage time between homework and family, organize your day, prevent meltdowns, catch up on failed projects, and so on.
- Whenever possible, hire outside help to do daily, necessary tasks such as cleaning the house, maintaining the lawn, and anything else related to the family's environment. A tidy home (in a normal way, not manic or even "magazine-like") reflects positively on the state of mind of those who live in it. If your family budget does not allow for outside help, consider swapping chores with friends, relatives, and neighbors. Ask relatives or friends to fill in for you by reciprocating with something you can do for them. For example, if you enjoy gardening but hate vacuuming, suggest to a friend that you fix the roses in her garden while she takes care of your floors in return.
- Take some time for yourself after work. Consider, for example, spending 20 minutes at a coffee house near your home or popping into a place you particularly like (a park, a museum, an interesting store...) to take your mind off things and get the energy back to give to your family.

- Set up quiet areas in your home to minimize distractions and sensory overload. Even a chair in the closet is fine, it is a bit funny, I know, but everyone does not need to know it is your place of silence, right?
- While I do not want to contradict the previous suggestion of keeping your home tidy, at the same time allow yourself to have "messy zones" at home so that there is not constant anxiety and frustration in trying to keep the entire house tidy. Make it a sort of island of escape.
- It is not easy, but, if possible, turn off the TV and especially the phone during meals.
- Have weekly family meetings to discuss problems and ways to solve them, this is where all filters should fall and there should be a calm and relaxed atmosphere, all family members should feel comfortable and free to express themselves.
- Find some healthy humor in the mishaps created by ADHD, laughing about it is sometimes the best therapy.
- Be prepared to have a plan for various situations. For example, if you know your child is always throwing tantrums at the grocery store, if possible, leave them at home with your spouse, a relative, or a babysitter.

- Find creative ways for the family to do chores, perhaps singing or dancing while passing the dust. Come up with contests to see who can finish a certain task first, offer weekly prizes, but do it all in a relaxed atmosphere. For example, if there are two children, you can invent that whoever finishes tidying up their room first will get an extra half hour watching cartoons,, avoid offering prizes out of context such as an expensive toy or other exaggerated things.
- Set up a large erasable board and a different colored marker for each family member, for sports or school schedules, chores, homework, and so on. Blue marker for the male, pink for the female, red for dad, yellow for mum and so on, everything must be quite simple and fun.
- Have a "dedicated place" for everyday items that are typically lost several times a day. This is usually keys, phone, earbuds, glasses, wallet. For example, take a pocket emptier and put it on a small table next to the entrance, decide that is where the keys will always be stored. All keys, so house keys, car keys, office keys, gym locker keys, etc., should be stored there.
- Prepare things ahead of time so there are no hectic moments before heading out to start the day. For example, the packed lunch is good to prepare it the night before, as well as clothes and possibly an

umbrella or what you know you may need the next day, put your briefcase and school folders next to the door where the family comes out.

- Put a small chalkboard or block notes on the refrigerator where family members can jot down food items to buy. For example, if one of the members finishes the last bottle of milk, they can write milk on the grocery list at the same time they finish it.

- Remind yourself and your family that ADHD is not a death sentence or something to be ashamed of and that, together, you will overcome these difficulties through humor, creativity and thinking outside the box.

- Follow the basics of a good lifestyle: exercise, good diet, and adequate sleep. Some people find that meditating is helpful for keeping calm and focused, or even listening to some nice and relaxing bedtime stories in audiobooks when it is time to sleep.

- Simplify meals if cooking is not your best talent. Allow yourself to plan dinners and use shortcuts to prepare tasty, yet quick and easy meals (for example, you can make cooking part of the favor exchanges mentioned earlier. If you have a neighbor or relative or friend who cooks well, you can exchange favors. She or he cooks for you and your family, you take care of tidying up the yard, walking the dog, picking up laundry from the laundry room, etc.). Many children with ADHD are very picky eaters and it is best not to fight the problem otherwise you could run into eating disorders or various deficiencies.

- Use checklists and other organization strategies such as smartphone reminders or a paper planner (the classic pen notes on the calendar just to name one example). Make sure the system works for you, rather than investing in the latest gadgets just because they are popular.
- Pick your battles and let go of the things that are not that important. For example, they are fighting at work to get a new coffee maker, but you hypothetically do not like coffee, then let it go. Do not get involved and feel bad if you do not take part in the issue.
- As a parent, be consistent with house rules and show a united front. Follow routines and create a comfortable atmosphere. Children, as well as adults, with ADHD thrive within structure.

Well, we all know that raising a family is challenging, it is challenging even under the best of circumstances. If you then add ADD or ADHD to the mix, the stress can affect everyone involved. It is important to recognize the special challenges these families face. Allow yourself to step back, change your expectations, and forgive yourself when you feel you are not doing a "good enough" job such that you are juggling family and work. Think of new strategies, starting with the ones mentioned above, to improve your family's daily life. Remember that if you have ADHD, it is not your fault, but on the other hand, it should not be an excuse for problems your family might encounter.

Recognize that you are doing the best you can and reward yourself where the results are really good. Nonetheless, you will most likely need outside help and support from the expertise of mental health professionals and to ensure domestic help in managing some of the chores when possible. Remember then to delegate household responsibilities, or have some sort of outside supervision, and most importantly never stop keeping a high sense of humor and getting the treatment needed for all members touched by ADHD.

Each family member brings a special uniqueness to the family. All members have talents and passions, strengths, and insights. Showing appreciation or advice regularly will help improve self-esteem and bring the family closer together. We often tend to shine the spotlight only on the negative points or weaknesses that plague people, but this only creates more family tension and resentment.

Your job as an ADHD or ADD parent, with kids with the same disorder and otherwise, is extremely challenging. Keep your sense of humor, your awareness, and a solid self-esteem, finally remind yourself that you are doing the best you can.

11. ADHD and Eating Disorders

Foods to avoid.

Is there a possible role for nutrition in the treatment of attention deficit hyperactivity disorder? The topic is controversial, yet more and more industry studies are focusing on the subject, as well as numerous articles and even specific profiles on social media appearing on various blogs.

The recent increase in interest in the use of specific nutrition as an alternative to drug therapy for ADHD makes this discussion increasingly relevant. In particularly the use of omega-3 supplements and the shift away from a Western style diet to counteract an industrial style diet. Diets to reduce symptoms associated with ADHD include limiting sugar, eliminating preservatives, elimination diets, and supplementation with omega-3 fatty acids.

Supplementation with omega-3 is the most recent nutritional treatment with positive reports of efficacy, while cyclically the preservative-free diet developed in the '70s makes a comeback, sometimes forgetting the obvious evolution that has taken place over time from the point of view of studying nutrients (until a few years ago there were still no ingredient labels applied to all foods on the market, just to give a practical example).

Foods potentially associated with ADHD include: all fast food, red and processed meat, chips and high-fat dairy products, sugary and energy drinks. Instead, fish, vegetables, tomatoes, fresh fruit (juices and smoothies are preferable to packaged fruit juices often rich in added sugar), whole grains and low-fat dairy products are preferred.

In general, however, the important thing is to prefer a diet and lifestyle as healthy and varied as possible, as already mentioned in the previous chapters, together with a good physical exercise. Because those with ADHD find it really difficult to regulate emotions and have poor impulse control, it is very easy to run into eating disorders. Eating is, after all, a very stimulating activity and can bring with it a certain sense of comfort. Many people with ADHD use food as a remedy to overcome or soothe anxiety, stress, anger, boredom and so on. It is extremely important, again, to seek the advice of an eating disorder expert who is also remarkably familiar with all aspects of ADHD.

Below I am going to list what are considered the foods that should be avoided in case of ADHD.

Gluten

In some research, gluten is directly related to ADHD in both children and adults. One study shows a significant improvement in behavior and tasks following the initiation of a gluten-free diet.

Therefore, researchers believe that Celiac Disease should be included in the ADHD symptom checklist. It is important to recognize, however, that many individuals have a gluten intolerance but do not have Celiac Disease, despite having some of the same symptoms.

For a diet to treat ADHD be sure to avoid all foods that contain gluten including, pasta, bread, cereals, and packaged foods. Instead, look for gluten-free alternatives that are now increasingly easy to find both in physical stores and online.

Sugars

Young people who consume sweetened or energy drinks are 66% more at risk for hyperactivity and attention deficit than those who do not use them. Researchers recommend that intake of these beverages be limited as much as possible or even avoided, especially in children. It is not only adolescents who should avoid sugary drinks, as sugar is associated with ADHD even in adulthood.

Therefore, everyone is encouraged to avoid highly concentrated forms of sugar, including non-fresh fruit juices, carbonated soft drinks, candies, desserts and all sweets in general (especially industrially produced ones).

Food colorants

Consumption of artificial food dyes has increased fivefold since 1950, showing that the average consumption is 68 milligrams. Studies that have tested as little as 50 milligrams have shown a correlation between the intake of artificial dyes and behavioral reactions such as hyperactivity.

Artificial food dyes are found in virtually every packaged food, including sodas, low-quality foods, deli meats and cheeses, cereals, chewable vitamins, and toothpastes. As part of the ADHD treatment diet, all of these foods should be avoided. One tip is to always read the labels carefully on the products you choose. Finally, try to find diversions to color foods such as using turmeric or saffron for yellow, beet for pink, squid ink for black and so on.

Artificial Sweeteners

Artificial sweeteners such as acesulfame K, aspartame, benzene, cyclamate, saccharin, and sucralose are related to a number of serious side effects: cancer, obesity, tachycardia, infertility, memory loss, headaches, and dizziness. Although removing sugars from the diet is satisfactory against ADHD symptoms, replacing them with artificial sweeteners is not the most appropriate solution. Instead, try to add flavor to your dishes through natural herbs, spices and citrus fruits while using natural sweeteners in extreme moderation.

Caffeine

A recent study indicates that alcohol and caffeine consumption is associated with anger and violence in adolescents. Therefore, along with adults, adolescents with ADHD should avoid energy drinks with a high concentration of sugar, caffeine, and other stimulants.

While some prescription stimulants are indicated for the treatment of some cases of ADHD, it is imperative that all forms of caffeine (thus including beverages that contain some percentage of it) be removed within the diet, considering that it also increases anxiety, insomnia, and other symptoms.

If you just cannot give up coffee, for example in the morning, limit the consumption to a maximum of one coffee per day in minimum doses (the ideal is to learn to stop after a few sips).

Conventional Dairy

A 10-week study found that removing cow's milk from the diets of hyperactive children caused effective improvement in ADHD symptoms. The diet also eliminated artificial colors and flavors, chocolate, MSG, and caffeine.

Should some ADHD symptoms appear after consuming dairy products, it would be wise to remove them from one's diet. The most common cow's milk contains the protein casein A1, which can trigger a gluten-like reaction and therefore should be eliminated from the diet in both adults and children. Raw milk, which therefore has not undergone any thermal process, may be more appropriate for those with ADHD due to its immune-boosting properties. Goat's milk can also be considered an excellent substitute to classic cow's milk, as it does not contain A1 casein.

Remedy Omega 3 and 6 deficiencies

The importance of omega-3, omega-6 is due to their fundamental role in brain function as well as in normal growth and development.

Too often for adults it is not easy to integrate these substances enough, even though it is recommended to eat more foods such as cold-water salmon, mackerel, anchovies, avocado, winter squash, cold pressed olive oil, walnuts, almonds (this is not the place to analyze each nutrient, but I suggest you do some research on which foods contain more sources of omega 3 and 6).

There is also an alternative solution from a supplementation standpoint, which is evening primrose oil. This completely vegetable oil is rich in essential fatty acids that provide the building material for cell membranes and a whole series of hormones or chemicals that mimic their effects. The intake of evening primrose oil is recommended in the form of a supplement, just to ensure compliance with the composition and safety.

Nitrites

Nitrites are chemical compounds derived from nitrous acid, consisting of one nitrogen atom and two oxygen atoms. They are mainly found in cold cuts and sausages, fresh cooked or seasoned, smoked, and canned meats, canned goods subjected to sterilization. Most packaged and canned foods contain Nitrites. They cause restlessness and anxiety that can worsen ADHD symptoms. In addition, Nitrites in the diet are related to an increased risk of developing type 1 diabetes, certain types of cancer, and irritable bowel syndrome.

12. Practice Mindfulness Meditation in ADHD

Several studies have shown how complementary therapies of alternative medicine have an important role in the treatment of the disorder. Mind-body therapies, in fact, are the most widely used and among them include approaches based on Mindfulness and meditation have a significant impact on psychosocial, emotional, and neurobiological functioning. These techniques use deep breathing or meditation, seek to expand the field of awareness using guided visualization, progressive relaxation, and simple yoga exercises. It has been shown that the practice of these therapies can significantly help improve mood and reduce anxiety, stress, and pain, as well as develop control of attention, awareness and regain one's inner balance.

Considering these benefits, some intervention studies have applied Mindfulness Meditation for the purpose of controlling ADHD symptoms in children and adolescents, across all subtypes, and even in adults. In particular, the greatest effects are seen on inattention, hyperactivity or impulsivity and related abilities such as accuracy speed and reaction time. Other secondary results are related to anxiety, shyness, social problems, and perfectionism as well as acting on emotional dysregulation and possible depressive symptoms. These results are important because they identify the positive and multidimensional fallout of complementary interventions compared to, for example, pharmacotherapy, which is often correlated with side effects such as poor tolerance, no response to treatment, and even dangerous dependence.

So, what is Mindfulness Meditation?

Mindfulness Meditation is a practice based on the awareness of the present you are living and on the importance of paying attention to yourself in every moment of the day. Only when you are truly attentive you can listen, understand, and live reality in a more serene way, curbing that latent and perennial inner suffering until you reach a complete acceptance of yourself. Therefore, the combination of Mindfulness and ADHD could lead to amazing results.

When you meditate to achieve your mindfulness, you do not need to be looking for specific benefits, you just need to focus exclusively on the practice, because that is the only way we can train the mind to be focused on the present. In essence, the positive effects of this technique are many: when we are mindful, we reduce our stress levels, we increase our performance, we know how to evaluate situations with a more critical eye, and we increase our attention towards the well-being of ourselves and others.

Mindfulness meditation gives those who practice it moments in which it is possible to suspend judgment and tap into our natural curiosity about how the mind works, approaching our experience with warmth and kindness towards ourselves and others.

Mindfulness, like some of its other "cousins", is a type of meditation that can be performed at any time of day. In the early days, especially in those who have a certain diagnosis of ADHD, it is recommended to practice it in small moments of pause between commitments, or for example in the shower, while you are in the waiting room maybe the dentist or hairdresser, or on the train during the journey home. Start with small moments in which you clear your mind to get back into it, with time it will become easier to do this even while performing other actions.

Some types of meditation need a lot of practice before allowing practitioners to reach a level advanced enough to show tangible benefits on the well-being of body and spirit. Mindfulness is, on the other hand, remarkably simple. Mindfulness is always available to us.

Therefore, as already anticipated, it is recommended for those with ADHD of any kind to stop as soon as you have a moment or think about meditation or remember, breathe slowly, and ask yourself questions about your condition: What am I feeling right now and how intense is this feeling? How am I reacting to this situation?

As your mind absorbs these questions, it will be automatic to feel more aware of your current situation. It is also extremely useful to start paying attention to the body's impulses: feel the warmth of a sunbeam on your skin, observe (and not just look at) your surroundings, actively appreciate the smells that invade your nostrils. Logically, for a person with ADHD all of this could be extremely difficult and, in some ways, "disastrous", given the ease of distraction typical of the disorder, but with a lot of practice and good you will power, everyone could be able to obtain excellent effects. In a nutshell, the mission is to live a single moment with attention and self-awareness.

Although Western psychology is still particularly skeptical when it comes to meditation, many studies have reported that a more "mindfulness" life allow anyone, even those with ADHD, to reap clear benefits for your body and your mental health.

Many psychologists have integrated these techniques into a complex psychotherapeutic course in a way that complements classical therapy.

Dedicating a few minutes to this practice, in fact, you can see an increase in the activity of the prefrontal cerebral cortex where positive emotions reside and a neuro-modulated intervention on the axes of the pituitary gland and the secretion of cortisol. All this results in a regulation of emotions, greater concentration, a sense of calm, greater relaxation of the body and improved sleep quality.

Meditation in any case helps to keep the mind healthy, prevent disease, make people happier, and improve performance in virtually any task, be it physical or mental.

Since people with ADHD often also tend to do the opposite of distracting themselves, i in other words, hyper-concentrate, or hyper focus, all the more reason why an exercise in mindfulness and managing one's inner balance is not to be underestimated.

However, in order to experience most of these benefits you need to practice meditation consistently (every day).

The advice is to rely on professionals or consult specific and easy to understand texts to deepen the practice.

13. ADHD and Managing Finances

The problem related to poor impulse control and a known and established tendency to shop uncontrollably has already been mentioned several times in previous chapters. There is no shortage of evidence of people with ADHD who have bought the same objects several times because they had forgotten they already had them, or because they were convinced, they could not do without another similar product, or simply out of distraction. With ecommerce this phenomenon is highly amplified, there is no shortage of episodes of orders made at times when one was about to have a meltdown, or purchases made absent-mindedly while the site cart was already loaded with other products that one had forgotten to eliminate or loaded two or three times.

Adults with ADHD often have difficulty managing their money, paying bills, and meeting their debts or deadlines. Impulsivity, when still present in the adult, creates difficulty in delaying gratification, thinking, and planning for the future, which has a negative impact on managing their finances well. Forgetting to pay a bill can result in penalties, power cuts, problematic situations that then require effort and time to fix. In the same way, people with ADHD end up wasting money on impulse purchases of unnecessary items and products, food that expires or is forgotten to be consumed, clothes or gifts that are forgotten to pick up from the laundry or delivered to the right person. All this, in mild forms, can bring a smile to your face. Who has never succumbed to the temptation of buying an accessory or a discounted product on the wave of enthusiasm, and then regret it once you get home? But in the case of a person with ADHD, there is little to smile about. Hoarding items that one has spent little or a lot of money on can, in the long run, translate into an overwhelming problem. Even starting lots of hobbies, something that may seem innocent and even positive on the surface, can become dramatic. Buying a guitar, signing up for an app with a subscription, buying books that you forget to read, buying a sewing class, gym outfits, bonsai trees and plants that you then do not care for, all translates over time into an irreparable waste of money.

These money management issues can sometimes even lead the adult with ADHD back to living in the parental home because they simply cannot make it financially on their own; at least not yet. Little, if any, use is made of gimmicks such as taking away a person's credit card, as in times of compulsive shopping they will still find a way around the problem. For example, they may have memorized the card number, or they may open a different online account in a few clicks, pay with their PayPal account for example or another alternative wallet. Rather useful are work papers or alarms that sound, perhaps shared with your partner or a trusted coach, as soon as you access an app that requires payment.

In any case, therefore the advice is always to seek help from a trusted person or a professional, it is extremely important to always keep a watchful eye.

There are many reasons why money management is difficult for ADHD individuals. Financial planning relies on many executive functioning skills. It requires organization, time management, planning, and prioritization, all of which are more difficult for a person with ADHD.

For children with ADHD, the challenges they face in doing homework can become the same challenges they will face once they become adults with money management.

It is important, especially in the case of adult parents of children with ADHD, to talk about and early start helps children and teens develop good habits, such as setting spending limits and resisting impulse purchases.

Here are some tips and strategies that are useful at any age, and can help develop money management skills through routine activities:

- Setting a good example. The concept of money is learned primarily through the example of how others handles their money. Of course, for children, the point of reference is the parents and relatives.
- Set a small weekly allowance, with a clear understanding of what activities the money can be

allocated to. The child will learn that he or she will have to wait until next week before he or she can buy what he or she wants, and this will project into the monthly stipend he or she will receive as an adult.

- Allow money to be earned through household chores. Children should normally do these chores as members of the family, but for some in particular, it may be a way to allow them to earn some money to add to their tips. This teaches them that if you work for something you can receive a reward.
- Create structure for their money. Children, sometimes also adults, with ADHD benefit from structured environments in all aspects of their lives. This is equally true when it comes to money. In addition to agreeing on how they can spend their money, you can also teach them not to spend some of it (savings). All of this should be addressed as an adult with their family, coach or personal financial advisor.
- Help them plan ahead for their spending. Individuals with ADHD have issues with planning that extend to money. Because they prefer immediate rewards, and have trouble waiting for a bigger reward at a later time, it will be important to encourage them to wait instead of buying impulsively.

Money management involves developing a process of learning and awareness. Children with ADHD face more challenges while growing up than their peers, but with targeted help they can achieve good results for future adult life. Where help or a proper diagnosis has not been made in childhood, intervention in adulthood will be even more significant and necessary.

14. Strategies for Maintaining Focus If You Have ADHD

Although ADHD (attention deficit hyperactivity disorder) is often the target of jokes and humorous banter, for those with the disorder trying to focus on an important task can be anything but fun. Fortunately, mild to moderate ADHD symptoms can be kept in check through behaviors and mental strategies that help improve focus and attention. Let's continue this chapter to find out more.

Move constantly.

Have you ever seen someone who cannot stop shaking a leg, fiddling with a pen, a ring on a finger, fix an earring on the earlobe or doing some other kind of repetitive movement while trying to focus on something? If the answer is yes, you have observed a good example of what it means to move all the time. In short, we are talking about those repetitive physical movements that sometimes prove helpful in increasing concentration, especially for activities that require constant attention for long periods of time. For example, many students play with pencils or make small doodles on a paper while listening to a lecture, and this prevents them from drooping their eyelids and reconciling a state of boredom or sleep.

Of course, you should always take into consideration the circumstance in which you find yourself. If you work in a noticeably quiet office, for example, obviously it will not be appropriate to drum a pencil on your desk or over drum your fingers.

Keep your work area clean and clear.

Having a dirty desk is not only contrary to Feng shui. It can also be a major impediment to your ability to concentrate. Several studies have shown that a cluttered workspace, whether in the office or at home, decreases concentration. If there are several items that grab your attention, your brain will have to strain to spread it out among all of them, instead of focusing on the most important one (like the to-do list of emails in front of you). So, in a battle against distraction, a good solution is to get in the habit of cleaning up your work area before diving into an important task.

Try listening to soft music while you work.

Many people prefer to work while listening to music (mostly soft music, with no singing and no overly excited rhythms), and this includes people with ADHD. However, some recent research has shown that listening to music can increase activity in an area of the brain called the "default brain network" that is partly responsible for controlling how prone you are to being distracted by external stimuli.

Keep in mind that there is one important condition for this method to work: you must like the music you listen to. Listening to music you do not like has not been shown to have any effect on maintaining concentration, on the contrary it can only create tension and irritability.

Try talking to someone about your work.

Discussing the important things, or simply what you need to do, with other people can help you get on board and get the job done in a number of ways. First of all, talking about your tasks can help you understand them better. Kind of like when saying things out loud makes them seem clearer and "real". Since, in order to explain to someone else that you have to do something, you have to "digest" your task and break it down into its essential elements, this can be very helpful to you in understanding it better.

In fact, one of the strategies for dealing with ADHD is to tell someone that you will call or text them when you finish an important task. That way, that person will deem you trustworthy. If you beat around the bush and he (or she) does not hear from you, he or she will pressure you to finish the job.

Some people with ADHD finds it helpful to work or do homework in the presence of someone they care about, such as a family member or close friend. This way they can ask for help in maintaining focus or getting a clear understanding of what they need to do when their attention level drops. It is a kind of teamwork that can have surprising effects. However, if you find that you spend more time chatting and shooting the breeze than working when you have someone around, this method is not for you.

Make a to-do list.

The suggestion related to making a list I think is the most popular one ever in relation to ADHD. This is because sometimes just having the list of things you need to do in front of you, is motivation enough to start doing them. Having an organized and sensible list of missions makes it easier to tackle all the tasks of the day. Checking off things as you go along gives you a sense of accomplishment that will prompt you to continue immediately, without distraction. For people with ADD who have trouble remembering their important responsibilities, a to-do list can be an important incentive essentially because it helps keep things from being forgotten. If this method works, consider carrying a notepad or notebook with you, or use phone notes, so that you always have the list handy.

Make a clear and precise schedule for the day.

This is also one of the most popular strategies of all and has already been mentioned in the previous chapters. If you force yourself to follow a detailed schedule, it will be difficult to neglect important activities because you will automatically avoid situations where it is easy to incur distractions. Having smartphones and laptops at your disposal, by the way, makes it even easier to plan your schedule. Putting alarms on your phone to wake up, to remember to go to an appointment, a meeting, becomes essential. Logically, you have to maintain a certain consistency with the schedule, otherwise it will be useless.

Below I have sketched out a generic example that you might be inspired by; this schedule is designed for one weekday of a person who works full time, so feel free to modify it according to your needs and clearly depending on the type of work and lifestyle you deal (the day of a clerk will be of course very different from that of a bartender or a mason, a boutique saleswoman or a personal trainer or a housewife).

7:00: Wake up, take a shower and a healthy breakfast.

8:00: Leave the house to go to work.

8:15: Take the train.

9:00 a.m. - 12:00 p.m.: Focus only on the employment to be done as scheduled in the agenda. No distractions.

12:00 - 1:00 p.m.: Have lunch and then take a 20-minute walk outside in the fresh air, even if it's winter time.

1:00 p.m. - 5:00 p.m.: Focus only on the work to be done as planned in the agenda. No distractions. If anything, you can take a snack break (perhaps by taking one of the foods suggested in the previous chapter on the ideal diet for those with ADHD).

5:45 p.m.: Return to home.

6:00 p.m.: Free time (unless you have something important to do).

6:00 p.m. - 8:00 p.m.: Dinner.

8:00 - 11:00 p.m.: Free time (unless you have something important to do, but it would be better to unplug your mind and just relax).

11:00 p.m.: Bedtime.

Adopt healthy habits.

Although I know I am repeating things that have already been said, lifestyle can greatly affect concentration. Not being able to maintain focus on a task can become a big problem if it gets out of control, so increase your chances of success by following these simple tips.

Exercising is not only important for overall health, but it also helps when it comes to focus. Several research studies have shown that the right amount of exercise can increase your ability to maintain focus and brain activity.

Reduce caffeine consumption, please let me repeat. Despite the fact that caffeine is a stimulant and can therefore enhance certain cognitive functions (such as memory, concentration, etc.), it is not recommended at high dosages (you should not exceed 400 mg) for those with ADHD. Over time, caffeine consumption can lead to addiction accompanied by nervousness, headaches, and irritability, all of which make it even harder to focus on anything. In addition, caffeine can cause insomnia, and getting a good night's sleep is especially important for those with ADHD. If you want to know how to use caffeine if you are diagnosed with ADHD, consult your doctor to find out what the right dose is for your needs, concerning to your lifestyle, health status, and build.

Get enough sleep. It is already hard to concentrate with ADHD, without needing to add fatigue to it. Most adults need 7-9 hours of sleep to perform at their best; children need more. Since there is evidence that sleep disturbances are much more common in people with ADHD, good sleep care should not be underestimated at all.

Be aware of your attention spans.

The first step in mentally controlling ADHD symptoms is to identify them as soon as they appear. It has already been stated several times in the previous chapters how important it is to gain a good level of awareness. When you realize that you are starting to lose focus, or worse to have a moment of meltdown, you can use one of the mental techniques described in this section to regain control. It is easier to get back on track if you notice right away that you're getting distracted, so pay attention to these signs that warn you that your attention is waning:

- You start thinking about what you are going to do when you finish what you are doing.
- You focus more on your physical movements (drumming your fingers, etc.) than on the important task at hand.
- You worry about the things around you and no longer pay attention to what you must complete.
- You start daydreaming or thinking about things that have nothing to do with the employment you are doing.
- You repeatedly check your phone for notifications or log into a social network.

Use a mantra to stay focused.

Believe it or not, many people with ADHD find it helpful to repeat a motivational formula to focus or a "mantra" when they notice their attention waning.

The mantra can be a simple command to stay focused, such as "Finish your email. Finish the email. Finish the email....". But also, a simple "Do it, mate". There is no "right" way to use a mantra, the important thing is that it is positive and helps you affirm yourself, so feel free to experiment. A small prayer is also fine, or for example you could mentally repeat to yourself why you need or want to stay focused on your work, "Work hard to earn the money for that trip to Europe", "Work hard to buy a bigger house", "Work hard to ... " and so on.

Consult a doctor before starting any type of treatment.

Attention deficit hyperactivity disorder is a medical condition, not a sign of mental weakness or a personal problem. For this reason, if your ADHD symptoms are serious enough insurmountable that the DIY methods listed above do not work, your next step is to see a doctor or explain your difficulties in more detail to your attending professional.

Only a professional can make an accurate diagnosis of ADHD and decide what the best treatment is, also and of course based on your personal ADHD type and history.

15. Myths to Dispel About Women And ADHD

There are some myths to dispel about women and ADHD. The myth of myths is that girls cannot suffer from it. Yes, I heard this sentence many times unfortunately.

Women's ADHD is under-diagnosed and under-treated, they face different risks than men's ADHD, and they also present with a different range of symptoms. It has taken a long time and many specific studies, tests, and testimonies, to understand how attention deficit hyperactivity disorder occurs in girls and women and what problems it can create the purpose of this article and understand and outline the phenomenological differences in order to avoid the risk of missed diagnosis.

The risks and toll of suffering that can result from attention deficit hyperactivity disorder, on the other hand, are enormous for an adult woman, with remarkably high incidences of frustration on the part of the females involved. Yet despite over a century of research and thousands of published studies, ADHD remains largely misunderstood, this is especially worse when it comes to declining ADHD in the feminine.

The presence of the disorder in women, chronic in adulthood, has a phenomenology that is at times opposite and almost contradictory to that which we are accustomed to seeing in the male population. This diversity leads to a diagnostic misrecognition and a lack of understanding of the disorder. Knowledge of ADHD in women is still limited as few studies have been conducted on this part of the population.

For many years it was thought that attention deficit hyperactivity disorder (ADHD) was a problem only for boys. However, there are many researches that have identified a percentage of girls with ADHD, although at a much lower rate than that of boys. The reason for this gender-related difference remained obscure and unexplored until a few years ago. In fact, it seems that this difficulty in diagnosis is closely related to official diagnostic criteria.

Typically, women come to recognize their ADHD after one of their children has been diagnosed. As they learn more about ADHD, they begin to re-see, analyze, understand that some traits, some difficulties they experienced as girls and still experience, albeit in different ways, are attributable to ADHD.

"Girls with ADHD remain an enigma, often overlooked, misunderstood, and much debated," says Ellen Littman, one of the first psychologists and researchers to focus on gender differences in ADHD and advocate for a reexamination of the functional definition of the disorder. Littman theorizes that girls with ADHD are not identified and helped from childhood because male-descended models of the condition have been overrepresented in the literature.

One reason ADHD is not diagnosed in women is to believe that their symptoms are merely the result of hormonal imbalances or factors. Taking into account that PMDD (Premenstrual Dysphoric Disorder) is a terrible condition that involves fear, isolation, loneliness and other symptoms such as suicidal thoughts, anxiety or uncontrollable anger and crying episodes that are often almost unbearable, one can well imagine how difficult it can be to deal with everything while also having to manage one's own ADHD problem. ADHD is a condition that, as addressed in previous chapters, can be extremely destructive to people's lives. Those with it often say that their lives are characterized by poor performance, frustration, and confusion about why things seem so difficult. A diagnosis can significantly improve things, but there are very few experts in treating this disorder in adult women. As a result, most clinicians use standard approaches that often do not help a woman with ADHD learn how to better manage her daily life.

ADHD-focused therapies are being developed to address a wide range of issues including self-esteem, interpersonal and family problems, daily habits, daily stress levels, and coping skills. Such interventions are often referred to as "neurocognitive psychotherapy," which focuses on life management skills to improve cognitive function (remembering, reasoning, understanding, problem solving, evaluating, and using judgment), learn compensatory strategies, and restructure the environment.

Medication issues are often more complicated for women with ADHD than for men. Any pharmacological approach must consider all aspects of the woman's life, with attention to hormonal biological conditions, menstrual cycle, pregnancy, menopause, with an increase in ADHD symptoms whenever estrogen levels decrease women with ADHD are more likely to suffer from anxiety and/or depression as well as the tendency to substance addictions but also sentimental (so-called toxic relationships).

Not all girls with ADHD will have problems with addiction or risky behavior. Many of them will manage to have a "normal" life, although with considerable effort and thanks to the help of valid professionals, aggravated by cultural models that are still pressing and rigid today. Therefore, it is extremely important that anyone who knows they are dealing with an adult woman with ADHD be especially attentive, patient and present for that special person.

16. The Positive Side Of ADHD: Creativity

When we talk about any kind of disorder, we immediately think that it is a condition with solely negative and dramatic aspects. However, this is not always the case. Although disorders have several characteristics that cause difficulties and problems, they also have a positive side. ADHD, Attention Deficit Hyperactivity Disorder, which is being diagnosed more and more often, can be a clear example of this.

Disorder is not synonymous with illness. A syndrome does not define who we are. In fact, it is not the same to say, "a depressed person" and "a depressive person." Disorder is different from symptoms. Therefore, although it may seem hard to believe, there is a positive side to ADHD that can change our minds about this lack of attention, inability to complete a task, or impulsivity that we always consider negative.

Who thinks that lack of attention and inability to complete a task are completely negative aspects? Maybe they are, but in all this it is honest to notice the strong presence of creativity. Right often those with a diagnosed ADHD disorder act spontaneously, exploring everything around him or her and focusing on those details that, to others, are insignificant.

Even as children, those with ADHD look for different ways to entertain themselves. Some of these are very curious and original, the result of creative ability. If you notice, moreover, children with ADHD always try to experiment, to search on their own. In this regard, they are very independent. Perhaps the worst aspect is the frustration they feel when they are "forced" to sit still, "behave", not explore around them, and not loosen the reins of their incredible creativity. This bores them, makes them nervous and can be the cause of negative reactions. For this reason, if a child with ADHD likes to do something, it is critical that they do it. It is true that, very often, they do not follow the rules and don't do things as they should, but if something makes them happy, it will stimulate their creativity and help them to be enthusiastic youngsters, in the broadest meaning of the word.

What happens to us as adults?

When we go through a negative experience, we worry, sometimes we blame ourselves, and sometimes we feel hurt for a long time... On more than one occasion, we even hold a lot of resentment. This does not happen to children who suffer from ADHD and sometimes you can retain even as adults. This way of dealing with the most difficult situations can be incredibly positive for their future. Unlike those who do not suffer from this syndrome, in fact, children with ADHD manage to forget in a hurry and their world does not remain anchored to the circumstances that made them angry. This is due to the fact that they live in the present, but also because they tend to adapt to circumstances. Due to their rejection of boredom, of the same old days that pass one after the other, children with ADHD welcome with open arms all the new things that may come into their lives, even if they are not all positive. Relating this excellent tendency to adult life is more complex, but it can happen, and it is greatly beneficial.

For children with ADHD, even children of parents with ADHD, a last-minute change of plans, a move, or a circumstance that forces them down a certain path in their lives will never be a drama. This ability to adapt and forget is a trait that would be helpful for many adults to avoid unnecessary worry.

Many individuals with ADHD are incredibly energetic. In fact, they are the ones who come up with new resolutions and new challenges with which to have fun with their friends. These individuals love having new experiences, observing, and contemplating differences as a source of fun and inspiration.

This energy sometimes results in impulsivity. In the case of children with ADHD, they do not think much before they act, they just do it. This behavior drives parents crazy, as they fail to see the most positive aspect of this impulsiveness: learning fast. Many times, a missed diagnosis leads to profoundly serious consequences of impulsivity in the adult, as we have already seen in previous chapters.

Earlier we were talking about boredom, but what happens when a person with ADHD does not like or care about something?

Children with ADHD focus all their energy on doing that specific activity. If they really like something and can do it, they will never put it off until tomorrow. This is not far removed from the behavior of the adult with ADHD.

Although we are used to seeing and analyzing disorders from a negative point of view, in reality, there are several that also have a positive side. We just need to look at them from a different perspective to be able to enhance their positive aspects and tilt the scales in their favor.

17. A Direct and Moving Testimony

I found this very poignant testimony that tells the tenacious struggle of a woman to live with and mitigate in some way a disorder as pervasive as ADHD, and I thank her from the bottom of my heart for writing and sharing it.

I hope it moves you, at least as much as it moved me.

At the age of 38, I was diagnosed with ADHD.

Most people's lives are uphill, you know, it is not a discovery. You are born carefree, only to become more and more busy as your responsibilities grow. For me, it was the reverse.

My childhood was a constant struggle, not because I was not fed, clean, and well-dressed, but because my body and mind seemed to go it alone.

The list of sensations and factors that caused me irritability and discomfort was awfully long, from fabrics to noises to smells to internal sensations, including that constant urge to do that is characteristic of ADHD.

I was constantly immersed in a sort of "stream of consciousness", a thought similar to a dream where the images followed each other at a rapid pace, with a non-linear and certainly not rational trend. I speak of images, but in my case, they were visions with very blurred edges, with a massive verbal component. I do not talk to myself; I imagine conversations with others. It is my way of processing reality.

This tangle of thoughts kept me from following the conversations. Imagine the scene. In elementary school there were groups of girls talking about this and that. I would follow the conversation for the first few moments, then get lost. At some point I would be asked for an opinion, and I would piece together the first and last bits of conversation. Laughter and jeers. "What you said has nothing to do with it!"

Hyperactivity is also not how one imagines it. For me, it means having a constant sense of dissatisfaction even after days that are bursting at the seams, even if there is virtually no break in between activities, even if I am doing two or three things at once. Reading, eating, listening to music, talking on the phone, as long as it alleviated that feeling.

As a kid I read all the time, I reached the record of Donald Duck comics read and reread and reread. When I had some space I would run around, otherwise I would seek an escape wherever I could. If I did not have an escape, I became deeply restless and irritable and ended up picking fights with my parents.

I felt inferior to my parents. I remember that my mother had big, strong, precise hands. I had short, weak, wobbly hands. When we would argue she would remain almost impassive, at most she would have a puzzled or worried look on her face. I could not control myself. I would cry and scream for hours until I felt exhausted, then I would feel guilty.

Adolescence got better; I could finally help myself! I was doing well in school; I had my own strategy. I would study hours and hours, walking back and forth. The first years I had a few low grades, even failures, then I discovered the trick: I had to make the teachers understand that I was studying. I would never fail to memorize a detail from the textbook to show off in questions. It was my way of making it clear that if I did not know certain things, it was because I simply... did not remember them. I would also write down everything the professor said during class so that I would not have to rely on my memories. My nemesis was class assignments. Whispers and rustles would erase my thoughts in one fell swoop and I would have to pick up the thread again. I usually tacked something on the last hour, with my horrible handwriting full of erasures.

In my mid-20s, I had an eating disorder. I kept feeling inferior and wanted to do something to control myself, to get better. I thought I would control my eating to get to control my behavior: it did not work out that way.

I ended up feeling worse than before and it took several treatments, including medication, to get back to a decent balance. The ADHD meanwhile was there, undisturbed, and undiagnosed.

In the meantime, I made a life for myself. I changed jobs often, had no firm footing. I was always on the move, always restless. So, for years, between highs and lows, I became more and more adept at managing a way of being that now seemed unchanging. Couldn't I cooperate with other people? I did without. Could not build a career? I learned to save money.

A few months ago, I was diagnosed with ADHD. I started medication right away. It usually takes at least 4 weeks before you see the benefits. I saw them from the very first administration. I felt an easing of a feeling of constant muscle tension that I frankly thought was part of the human experience, instead it was just part of mine.

After a couple of months, I brought my son's face into focus for the first time. I cannot see well, despite wearing extraordinarily strong contact lenses with which I approach normal vision. Yet I do not see things. I do not observe them.

He also looked at me with an expression that alone is worth a lifetime. It was as if he were saying to me: "You've finally seen me mummy, you're finally there!". Oh, how much emotion I felt, and gratitude. Now I will continue to follow what the doctors tell me and try to live with ADHD by trying to have more and more awareness of the disorder day by day.

18. The 12 Most Famous Personalities With ADHD

There are many people affected by this disorder including a large number of well-known personalities.

For some it has been considered as an anomaly, but in other cases, given the difficulties they have had to face and overcome, it has allowed them to develop other types of characteristics such as greater creativity, even providing positive reinforcement to their personalities in the long run.

In this chapter we review 12 famous people who have suffered or are suffering from ADHD.

1. Simone Biles

It was the same American gymnast and Olympic champion who stated that she was already taking pharmaceutical drugs to treat ADHD since the age of 19. She was also found several times positive in doping tests because of her treatment.

This athlete represents the exception to the rule, teaching the world a profound lesson: even in a sport where extreme concentration and application is required, ADHD does not suppose a barrier to success.

2. Ryan Gosling

The famous Canadian actor, star of famous movies such as "Noa's Diary", "Drive" or "La La Land" has been living with ADHD since he was diagnosed during his childhood. A fact that caused him many problems during his school time because he could not read and that led him to suffer bullying episodes.

3. Sylvester Stallone

During his childhood, the iconic action movie actor and unforgettable performer of Rocky Balboa and Rambo, in their respective sagas, suffered several problematic episodes at school that led to his expulsion from more than 14 schools. He was a wild child and very restless due to ADHD. However, the disorder did not stop him from becoming a movie icon.

4. Michael Jordan

The most famous basketball player of all time has also suffered from ADHD since childhood. His hyperactivity reached the point that several doctors and teachers told his parents that he would not have great professional and work opportunities because of his obvious lack of concentration. Currently, he is considered one of the best athletes and champions in all of history.

5. Michael Phelps

He is the most successful Olympic athlete ever thanks to 28 medals won at the Olympic Games. The famous swimmer during a press conference said that during his teenage years he was diagnosed with ADHD. Despite being told by one of his teachers that he would never achieve anything important in his life, he used swimming as a therapy for his disorder and the results have gone down in world sports history.

6. Usain Bolt

Again, an athletic icon of the Olympics. The Jamaican sprinter is one of the most surprising cases. The world record holder had a difficult childhood because he was a very restless and hyperactive teenager, a fact that ended up influencing his upbringing. Again, ADHD was not an obstacle at all, managing to find his escape and expression in athletics and speed.

7. Bill Gates

The computer mogul, co-founder of Microsoft and one of the richest people in the world. From an early age, he was an intensely curious child who would not stop asking questions about anything that called his attention. Later, due to his lack of performance in studies because of ADHD, he was forced to drop out of Harvard University, which did not stop him from founding his own company and launching Windows in 1985.

8. Walt Disney

The famous creator of movies and animated characters we love so much was a boy who suffered from severe concentration problems. He preferred to spend his time drawing and daydreaming, which led him to be considered "weird" by many of his peers. He devoted himself to distributing newspapers, which ended up totally affecting his school performance. He was also fired from several jobs in communication and media because of the difficulties and distraction caused by his disorder.

9. Agatha Christie

The successful British mystery writer has been considered the "slowest" person in her family since childhood. Not only was she diagnosed with dyslexia, but also ADHD, and throughout her life she struggled with both disorders.

Despite having very bad handwriting, her works reached the whole world, and she became one of the most famous writers of all time.

10. Jennifer Lawrence

One of the highest paid young actresses in the world and to have had an Oscar for one of her performances. However, her childhood was far from easy: at school she was called "nitro" (nitroglycerin) for her constant hyperactivity before she was diagnosed with ADHD.

Lewis Hamilton

The British Formula 1 driver was the youngest person to win a World Cup, equaling Michael Schumacher as the most awarded driver in history with seven championships. Hamilton was a very restless and undisciplined child who was later diagnosed with ADHD. However, from the moment he drove his first kart at the age of six, it was immediately clear to him that he wanted to dedicate himself to the world of motor racing, and certainly his restlessness or lack of concentration in other areas did not stand in his way.

Final Thoughts

ADHD is an overwhelming, often exceedingly frustrating, and disruptive condition still too often questioned and misunderstood. People say whoever has ADHD is just needs to try harder, or get organized, or stop procrastinating.

Uh, if only it were that simple!

ADHD is not a nuance of personality.

Anyone who has ADHD knows it is a problem. A real, concrete problem, not a nuance of character or personality. It is ubiquitous and undeniable. It affects the entire existence in all its aspects and in the vast majority of cases brings with it other "nice disorders" such as insomnia, depression, anxiety, phobias of various sorts and a marked tendency to impulsivity. However, for almost anyone outside the brain of a person with this diagnosis, ADHD is a contradictory and confusing concept.

Those around people with ADHD often show off expressions that are perplexing to say the least, try to reconcile a marked creativity and incredible energy, which often make people fall in love with them, with distracted behavior and especially mood swings that are comparable to a roller coaster. Family, friends, and colleagues struggle to frame the person with ADHD. They wonder, "How could such an intelligent person be capable of such foolish choices?" "If you only wanted to, you could do it differently," they say.

But they do not. They do not know that this is not the case.

ADHD is a condition of contradictions.

Most of the traits of a person with ADHD reflect two extremes on one continuum. For example, it is extremely difficult for a person with ADHD to keep his or her focus on something that lasts a long time (a movie, a ceremony, a conversation, a lecture, a meeting, and so on), but at the same time he or she happens to hyper-focus on something (which can be either something he or she is normally excited about or can be a temporary interest generated by a trigger). In that moment of hyper focus, it may happen that the individual skips meals, forgets to have appointments, to turn on the phone... metaphorically he goes into another space-time dimension.

In a fraction of a second, an unstoppable shift occurs between disturbing distraction to extreme focus.

ADHD is a brain phenomenon.

Brain patterns with ADHD are difficult to decipher no matter what, but sometimes they are so complex that they are complicated even for the best professionals. And by "sometimes," you could say basically constantly.

In the ADHD brain, neurotransmitters in the areas that control attention are comparable to sloths, which seems counterintuitive since active minds are constantly moving like crazy balls.

This chemical imbalance confounds researchers, who suspect that the disorder is largely genetic in nature. But since there is no way to prove ADHD beyond a behavioral checklist and a handful of rating scales, it is even harder to believe.

Those around someone with ADHD recognize the differences in their brain chemistry.

These are people bombarded daily with insecurity and self-criticism, despite being aware (especially with an official diagnosis) that their behavior is not intentional but is driven by chemicals in the brain called neurotransmitters.

ADHD is a daily struggle.

Most people cannot comprehend the number and complexity of the daily challenges an individual with ADHD battles with themselves. The simplest tasks, such as picking up a dry cleaning or sending an email, can become impossible missions. A payment, a phone call, or an errand can suck up all their energy. Everyone clearly experiences their disorder in a more or less exhausting way, personal circumstances such as age, educational background, social and work expectations matter a lot, but for everyone it simply isn't easy.

Some might say, "Well, life isn't easy for anyone," and that is true. But to those who claim this, they should try living a single day in the mind of a person with ADHD and they would understand how exhausting and frustrating it can be to try to package a professional email while in their head they are playing a pinball league with lights balls splashing everywhere, bells, music, and whatnot.

Those same individuals with ADHD ask themselves, "I'm a person of great ability, I've even graduated from college and am successful in many areas of life, yet why can't I ever pay a bill on time?" The answer is rarely hidden in the task itself, but rather in a specific component that triggers something in the ADHD brain that shifts the focus. What shifts the attention might be an unhappy decision, a deadline, incomprehensible rules, or something so boring they can't stand it.

ADHD at arm's length with insecurity.

Most people could not tolerate the voices echoing in the head of an individual with ADHD. It can be helpful to imagine crowds of little sprites appearing a second after each action with a sign and the question: *"why did I say that? Did I make a bad impression? Why can't I ever get the job done on time? How could I be so forgetful? Why can't I stop buying unnecessary things?"*

This exhausting living with self-accusation makes individuals with ADHD their own harshest critics.

ADHD and the invisible effort.

People with ADHD really do try to put in the effort, as opposed to those who think they forget things out of disinterest or disregard or that they "just have their heads in the clouds."

All they would often need is a little patience, healthy non-judgmental affection, and understanding. If a huff and a roll of the eyes over the umpteenth time you could not find your keys or forgot an anniversary was replaced with a "come on, let us look for your keys together and decide on a place to always store them" or "don't worry, we'll celebrate this anniversary with the next one," the benefits would be much greater.

ADHD and relationships.

This truth may be the hardest for neurotypical spouses, parents, and managers to accept. ADHD is biologically woven into the DNA of the person diagnosed and never goes away (although it can be managed).

The best thing to do is to trust the person's attempts to curb ADHD and do your best to be there for them, whether it is a romantic partner, a friend, a co-worker, whoever.

ADHD and exponential emotions.

Whether it is anger, joy, worry, or whatever of something, an individual with ADHD feels all emotions as if they have an exponential factor. The emotions and the thoughts related to them are cumbersome and bursting with intensity. Often one encounters people with ADHD who fill or light up a room when they arrive, metaphorically speaking, and begin to speak in a logorrheic manner and with passionate urgency, sometimes anticipating answers to questions that have not yet been fully formulated. It also happens, however, that these same "hand grenades" thrown at full force are then a source of repentance and embarrassment for the person with ADHD.

ADHD is not a random excuse.

"I forgot to do this." "I'm trying my best" "I'm sorry." These may seem like quite common and rather trivial excuses or escape routes; they are not. Unfortunately, however, it is not always possible for an ADHD person to say, "*I messed up because of my ADHD.*" It is not an explanation that many people would understand, and it is especially not something that can be flaunted to the four winds. It is easy to assume that if a man can say such a phrase to his wife, the same cannot be done lightly with his superior at work (where perhaps he has just started). But the phrase contains the whole truth. ADHD is the reason why this people do what they do. It is frustrating to have a disorder that no one believes in. ADHD is illogical and extremely complicated to explain even for those who have it. So, it is even more delicate and critical that those on the other side of the fence offer mindful and patient support.

ADHD and who will change the world!

ADHD is the source of creative vision, courage, and incredible passion.

As already said, those with ADHD can have absolutely brilliant ideas, sometimes spawned from being able to see and observe things that normal minds do not see. They are able to come up with revolutionary inventions, perform extraordinary feats and have an unshakeable determination (see the chapter on famous personalities), which leads them to achieve fabulous successes in the most various fields. If managed properly, ADHD can be a hotbed of brilliant minds capable of changing the world.

Many exceptionally good and well-known authors at the end of their essays or manuals on ADHD have quoted Steve Jobs, and I too could not find a better quote to close this little text of strategies for adults, which I hope will bring serenity to the lives of those diagnosed with ADHD and, or even, to those who love them.

"Here are the crazy ones, the misfits, the rebels, the troublemakers, the round pegs in the square holes ... those who see things differently; they are not fond of rules and have no respect for the status quo.

They can self-criticize, disagree with themselves, glorify, or vilify, but the one thing you can't do is ignore them because they change things.

They push the human race forward, and while some may be seen as crazy, we see genius in them, because the people who are crazy enough to think they can change the world are the ones who do."

Thank you from the bottom of my heart for having chosen this book, I say goodbye wishing you the happy life everyone deserves.

This has been:

ADHD IN ADULTS

Effective Strategies, Skills, And Self-Help

To Improve the Quality of Life

For Those Who Have It

And Those Who Take Charge of a Loved One.

Written by **Diana Shelby**

Copyright **2021** by **Diana Shelby**

Production Copyright by **Diana Shelby**

www.ingramcontent.com/pod-product-compliance
Lightning Source LLC
Chambersburg PA
CBHW070650220526
45466CB00001B/368